Ageless Hormones

The Key to Lifelong Female Vitality

Ageless Hormones
The Key to Lifelong Female Vitality

What are the NoMAD Plans?

Developed by Dr Ash Kapoor, the NoMAD Plans represent a transformative approach to health and wellness that combines the wisdom of ancestral practices with contemporary medical insights. The name "NoMAD" not only suggests a journey through the intricate realm of health but also stands for its foundational principles: Nutritional Optimisation, Mindful Adaptation, and Detoxification.

At the heart of NoMAD is the 6R Framework—Restore, Release, Repair, Renew, Reframe, and Represent. This methodology addresses the root causes of illness, combats chronic inflammation, and cultivates authentic vitality, guiding individuals through a transformative process.

Tailored specifically to each individual, NoMAD journeys are meticulously crafted to rebalance the body, strengthen the mind, and rejuvenate overall health. By integrating ancestral practices with cutting-edge, innovative treatments—all under strict medical oversight—NoMAD Plans offer a personalised pathway to sustainable, long-lasting well-being that resonates with your unique life circumstances.

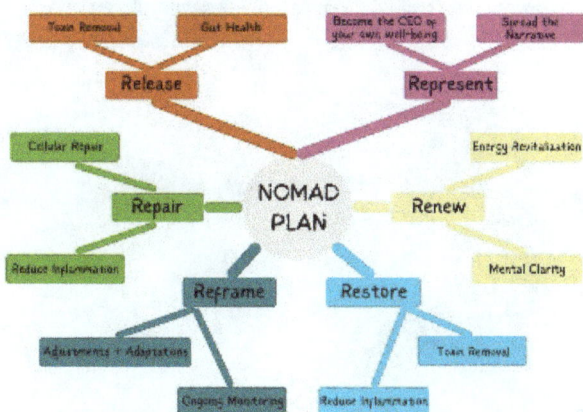

Levitas One:
"As Is In, As Is Out"

Reflecting the belief that our internal well-being is mirrored in our external environment. Founded by Dr. Ash Kapoor, Levitas One serves as the vehicle for delivering NoMAD's treatment plans. It envisions a healthcare future where patients are at the centre of a fully integrated, multidisciplinary approach. Guided by Nomads 6 Rs—Restore, Release, Repair, Renew, and Reframe, Represent—Levitas One empowers self-care through personalised guidance and minimal intervention, promoting long-term health, balance, and sustainability.

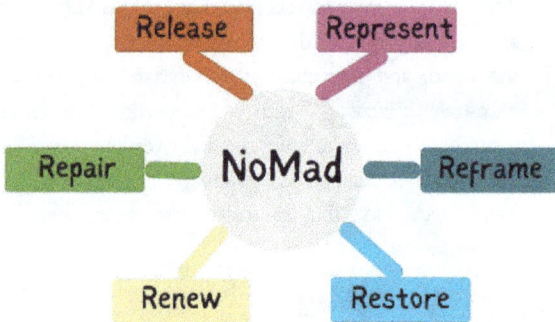

Contents

Preface

Over my 30-year career in medicine, specialising in hormone therapy, I have witnessed an incredible transformation in how we understand hormones and their role in our well-being. In this time, I have been privileged to treat thousands of women who have experienced the profound impact of hormone restoration on their health. Each of these women had her own unique journey, but one thing remained constant. When we worked to restore balance to their hormones, we also restored their vitality.

When I first started practising, hormone therapy was often seen as something only for menopausal women suffering from Hot flushes and night sweats. Today, we know that hormones are much more than just menopause management. They are the key to feeling energetic, youthful, and healthy at every stage of life. Whether you are in your 20s, 40s, or 70s, your hormones influence everything from your energy levels and mood to your bones, skin, and even your brain health.

What I have learned over the decades is that there is no "one-size-fits-all" approach to hormonal health. Hormones are dynamic and ever-changing, and each person's needs are unique. This is why personalised care is so critical. As a clinician, I have made it my mission to offer individualised solutions that suit each patient's body, lifestyle, and health goals. Whether it is Bioidentical Hormone Replacement Therapy (BHRT), nutrition, or lifestyle adjustments, my goal is always to find the right balance for each person.

Throughout my career, I have seen that when we take control of our hormones, we take control of our health. Women who have struggled for years with low energy, mood swings, poor sleep, or even severe menopausal symptoms often find a new lease on life when we get their hormones back in balance. For many, it is like turning the clock back—restoring their youth, confidence, and zest for life.

In this book, you will learn about the power of hormones and how you can use them to support your health at every age. You do not need to suffer from symptoms that are "just part of ageing." With the proper knowledge and the right support, you can enjoy vibrant health and energy well into your later years. I hope that by reading this book, you will feel empowered to take charge of your hormonal health and discover the incredible difference it can make in your life.

To your lifelong health and vitality,

Dr Ash Kapoor

Introduction

Why Hormones are the Key to Lifelong Female Vitality

Imagine your body as a well-run factory. In this factory, every system, every organ, and every process works in harmony to keep you feeling energetic, healthy, and youthful. But just like any factory, it needs someone in charge—managers to make sure things run smoothly. In your body, those managers are your hormones.

Hormones are the "master messengers" that control nearly every function in your body. They tell your cells when to create energy, when to burn fat, when to grow, and even when to rest. From the moment you wake up until you fall asleep, your hormones are at work behind the scenes, ensuring that your body operates as efficiently as possible. Whether it is your mood, your energy levels, your metabolism, or your reproductive health, hormones play a critical role in every aspect of your well-being.

Most of us think of hormones only when they become a problem—like during puberty, pregnancy, or menopause. But the truth is, hormones are always working in the background, affecting how we feel, how we look, and how we age. When your hormones are balanced, you feel vital and full of life. But when they are out of balance, you might feel tired, moody, or just not yourself.

This book delves into the world of hormones and their impact on your life from adolescence to your 70s and beyond. The goal is to empower you with knowledge about your hormonal health, enabling informed decisions about its support. Whether you are experiencing PMS, going through menopause, or seeking ways to maintain youthfulness and energy, this book provides the tools to take control of your hormonal balance for a more vibrant life.

What Are Hormones, and Why Are They So Important?

Hormones are chemical messengers that travel through your bloodstream, delivering instructions to your organs and tissues.

Produced by glands in your endocrine system—like the thyroid, adrenal glands, ovaries, and pancreas—hormones influence nearly every function in your body.

Think of them as the factory supervisors in your body. They oversee different departments, making sure each part of the factory (your body) knows what it needs to do, when to do it, and how much of it to do. For example, your thyroid hormones control your metabolism—the rate at which your body burns energy. Your sex hormones—like estrogen, progesterone, and testosterone—regulate everything from your menstrual cycle and fertility to your bone density and skin health. And cortisol, your stress hormone, helps you handle everything from daily stress to emergencies.

When everything is running smoothly, these hormones work together in harmony. But when one hormone gets out of balance—whether it is too much or too little—the entire system can feel off. That is when you start noticing symptoms like fatigue, weight gain, mood swings, or even more serious issues like infertility or osteoporosis.

The Factory Analogy: How Hormones Keep Your Body Running Smoothly

To make it easier to understand how hormones work, let us return to the idea of your body as a factory. Each system in your body—whether it is your digestive system, reproductive system, or immune system—has its own department. The hormones act as the managers, ensuring that everything stays on schedule and that all the systems communicate with each other.

For example:

- **Insulin,** produced by your pancreas, acts like a delivery truck, bringing sugar from your bloodstream into your cells for energy. Without enough insulin, your blood sugar stays too high, and you risk developing diabetes.

- **Estrogen** is like the quality control supervisor in women, ensuring proper function of your reproductive system and maintaining other important aspects of your health, like bone density and heart health.

- **Thyroid hormones,** like T3 and T4, are the speed regulators of your factory. They control how fast or slow your body's processes are running, from your metabolism to how quickly you use energy.

When everything is balanced, your factory runs like a well-oiled machine. But when one hormone is too high or too low, it is like a department manager not showing up to work. The other systems must work harder to compensate, and that is when things start to go wrong. You might feel constantly tired, gain weight despite eating well, or notice changes in your mood and sleep patterns. In short, hormonal imbalances can throw the whole system off.

Why Women Need to Pay Attention to Their Hormones

While hormones are essential for everyone, they play an especially crucial role in women's health. From puberty to pregnancy to menopause and beyond, a woman's hormonal needs change throughout her life. The fluctuations in hormones can cause a wide range of symptoms, from the minor annoyances of PMS to the life-altering effects of menopause.

Many women assume that these changes are just a part of getting older and that there is nothing they can do about it. But that is not true. The good news is that with proper knowledge and support, you can manage your hormones and keep them in balance throughout your life. This can help you not only feel better but also prevent long-term health issues like osteoporosis, heart disease, and cognitive decline.

Gain a deeper understanding of your hormones at every life stage. From your reproductive years to perimenopause and beyond, discover practical steps to optimise hormonal health and maintain vitality well into your 60s and beyond.

Empowering Women Through Knowledge: The Goal of This Book

The purpose here is simple: to give you the information you need to take control of your hormonal health. Too often, women feel powerless when it comes to their hormones, suffering through symptoms like fatigue, weight gain, and mood swings without knowing what is going on inside their bodies. I want to change that.

By understanding how your hormones work and what they need to stay balanced, you can make informed decisions about your health. This book will cover everything from the basics of hormone function to more advanced topics like Bioidentical Hormone Replacement Therapy (BHRT) and how lifestyle factors like nutrition, exercise, and stress management can support your hormonal health.

But this is not just about treating symptoms. It is about helping you live younger for longer. Your hormones play a crucial role in how you age, and by optimising them, you can maintain your energy, vitality, and overall health well into your later years. You do not have to accept that feeling tired, gaining weight, or losing interest in life is just a part of getting older. With the right approach, you can feel vibrant and full of life at any age.

What You will Learn in This Book

Here is a glimpse of what is ahead:

- **Chapter 1** will explore the basics of hormones—what they are, how they work, and why they are so crucial to your overall health.

- **Chapter 2** will dive into how hormones change during your reproductive years, from puberty to pregnancy and beyond.

- **Chapter 3** will guide you through perimenopause and menopause, offering practical advice on managing symptoms and debunking common myths about hormone therapy.

- **Chapter 4** will focus on Bioidentical Hormone Replacement Therapy (BHRT) and how it differs from traditional hormone therapy.

- **Chapter 5** will show you how to use hormones to support health and longevity, helping you live younger, longer.

- **Chapter 6** will look at natural ways to balance your hormones through diet, exercise, and stress management.

- **Chapter 7** will offer a decade-by-decade guide to navigating hormonal changes from your 20s to your 70s.

- **Chapter 8** will help you create a personalised hormone health plan to support you throughout your life.

- Finally, in **Chapter 9**, we will debunk myths surrounding the safety of critical hormones like DHEA, progesterone, estradiol, and testosterone.

By the end of this book, you will have a clear understanding of how hormones impact your health and what you can do to keep them in balance so you can live your best, healthiest life at every age.

Summary: Introduction

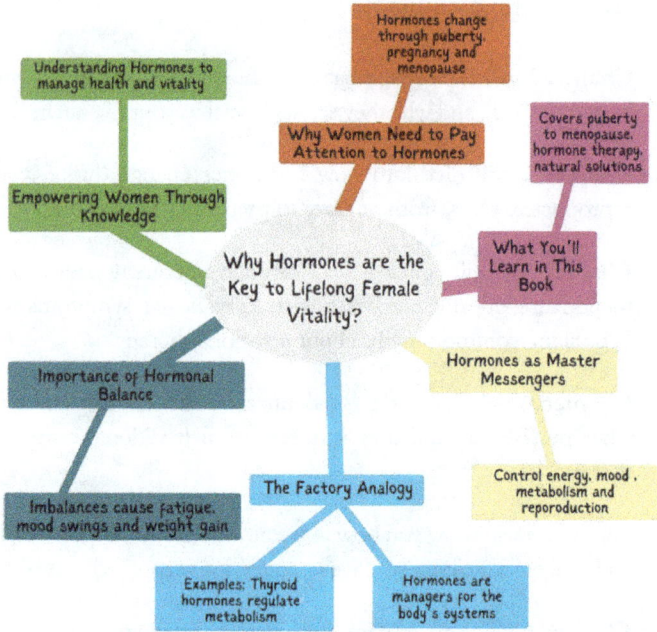

Hormones change through puberty, pregnancy and menopause

Understanding Hormones to manage health and vitality

Why Women Need to Pay Attention to Hormones

Covers puberty to menopause, hormone therapy, natural solutions

Empowering Women Through Knowledge

Why Hormones are the Key to Lifelong Female Vitality?

What You'll Learn in This Book

Hormones as Master Messengers

Importance of Hormonal Balance

The Factory Analogy

Control energy, mood, metabolism and reporoduction

Imbalances cause fatigue, mood swings and weight gain

Examples: Thyroid hormones regulate metabolism

Hormones are managers for the body's systems

Chapter 1
Hormones 101 –
What Are They and
Why Do They Matter?

Hormones. We hear the word all the time, often associated with mood swings, puberty, menopause, or fertility. But what are hormones, really? And why do they play such a crucial role in our health and well-being?

In this chapter, we will dive into the basics of hormones—what they are, how they work, and why they are so important for women at every stage of life. If you have ever wondered why you suddenly feel tired, gain weight, or experience emotional ups and downs, the answer often lies with your hormones. Understanding them is the first step to taking control of your health.

What Are Hormones?

Hormones are chemical messengers that travel through your bloodstream, delivering instructions to organs, tissues, and cells. They are produced by various glands in your body, which make up your endocrine system. This system is responsible for regulating everything from your metabolism and energy levels to your mood, sleep, and reproductive health.

Think of your body as a big company with many different departments. Your organs, tissues, and cells are like the employees, each with specific tasks to complete. But without clear communication, the whole company could fall into chaos. That is where hormones come in—they are the managers who pass instructions from the top down, ensuring that each department (or organ system) knows what it needs to do and when to do it.

For example:

- **Insulin**, produced by your pancreas, tells your cells to absorb sugar from your bloodstream, providing you with energy.

- **Estrogen** and **progesterone**, the primary female sex hormones, regulate your menstrual cycle, pregnancy, and menopause while also protecting your bones, skin and heart.

- **Thyroid hormones**, like T3 and T4, control your metabolism, influencing how fast or slow your body's systems work.

- **Cortisol**, your body's stress hormone, helps you manage both everyday stress and emergency situations by controlling blood pressure, inflammation, and energy production.

Each hormone has a specific job, but they do not work in isolation. They are part of an intricate network, constantly interacting with each other. When everything is balanced, this system works seamlessly. But if even one hormone is out of whack, the ripple effects can throw your entire body off balance.

The Endocrine System: The Hormone Headquarters

Your hormones are produced by glands that make up the **endocrine system**. This system is like the headquarters of a well-organised factory, with each gland responsible for producing different hormones.

Here is a quick look at some of the key players in your endocrine system:

1. **The Pituitary Gland** – Often called the "master gland," it controls other glands in your body, including the thyroid, adrenal glands, and reproductive organs. It secretes hormones like **growth hormone** and **luteinising hormone** (LH), which trigger ovulation and support reproductive health.

2. **The Thyroid Gland** – Located in your neck, the thyroid produces hormones that regulate metabolism, energy, and body

temperature. If your thyroid hormones are too low, you may feel sluggish and gain weight, while too much can leave you jittery and anxious.

3. **The Adrenal Glands** – Sitting on top of your kidneys, these glands produce **cortisol** and **adrenaline**. These hormones help you respond to stress. They also produce **DHEA**, a hormone that helps support your immune system and overall energy levels.

4. **The Ovaries** – These produce **estrogen** and **progesterone**, which are vital for reproductive health, bone density, and mood regulation. These hormones fluctuate throughout your menstrual cycle, pregnancy, and menopause, affecting everything from your skin to your sleep.

5. **The Pancreas** – This gland produces **insulin**, which helps regulate blood sugar. If insulin is out of balance, it can lead to serious conditions like diabetes.

These glands may be small, but they have an enormous impact on your health. They release hormones into your bloodstream, where they travel to specific tissues and organs, delivering the messages that keep your body running smoothly.

How Hormones Affect Your Body and Mind

Hormones have a profound impact on both your physical and emotional health. Here are just a few of the ways they influence your body and mind:

-   **Energy Levels** – Hormones like thyroid hormones and cortisol regulate how much energy your body produces and how efficiently it uses that energy. If these hormones are out of balance, you may feel tired or sluggish, even if you are getting plenty of sleep and eating well.

-   **Mood** – Hormones like estrogen, progesterone, and serotonin (a neurotransmitter influenced by your hormones) affect your mood and emotional well-being. That is why many women experience mood swings before their period (PMS), during pregnancy, or as they approach menopause. When hormone levels fluctuate, it can lead to feelings of anxiety, irritability, or even depression.

- **Metabolism and Weight** – Hormones like **insulin, leptin**, and **ghrelin** regulate your metabolism, appetite, and how your body stores fat. An imbalance in these hormones can make it harder to lose weight or control cravings, even if you are eating healthy and exercising regularly.

- **Reproductive Health** – From puberty through menopause, hormones like **estrogen**, **progesterone**, **FSH** (follicle-stimulating hormone), and **LH** control your menstrual cycle, fertility, and pregnancy. Changes in these hormones can affect everything from your ability to conceive to the severity of PMS or menopause symptoms.

- **Bone and Muscle Health** – Estrogen and testosterone help maintain bone density and muscle strength. As you age and hormone levels decline, you may experience a loss of muscle mass or a higher risk of osteoporosis, which is why it is so important to support your hormonal health throughout life.

- **Sleep** – Hormones like **melatonin** and **cortisol** regulate your sleep-wake cycle, influencing how easily you fall asleep and how rested you feel when you wake up. Hormonal imbalances can lead to sleep disturbances, insomnia, or feeling tired even after a full night's sleep.

The Impact of Hormonal Imbalance

What happens when your hormones are out of balance? Because hormones affect so many different systems in the body, the symptoms of hormonal imbalance can vary widely, but here are some of the most common:

- **Fatigue** – If you are feeling tired all the time, even after a good night's sleep, your thyroid or adrenal hormones might be to blame.

- **Weight Gain or Difficulty Losing Weight** – Hormones like insulin and thyroid hormones regulate your metabolism, and imbalances can make it hard to maintain a healthy weight.

- **Mood Swings** – If you find yourself experiencing irritability, anxiety, or depression, fluctuating estrogen or progesterone levels might be the culprit.

- **Irregular Periods** – An imbalance in estrogen or progesterone can cause changes in your menstrual cycle, from heavy periods to missed ones.

- **Low Libido** – Testosterone is not just for men—it plays a crucial role in sexual health for women too. A drop in testosterone can lower your libido and make sex less enjoyable.

- **Poor Sleep** – Cortisol and melatonin work together to regulate your sleep. If they are not in balance, you might have trouble falling asleep or staying asleep.

- **Hair Loss or Thinning** – Hormonal changes, particularly in estrogen and testosterone, can lead to hair thinning or loss, especially around menopause.

The good news is that once you understand what is causing these imbalances, you can take steps to address them.

Balancing Hormones: It is All About Communication

Balancing your hormones is a bit like maintaining communication in that factory we mentioned earlier. If one manager is missing or giving the wrong instructions, the whole system can fall apart. But when communication is clear and consistent, everything runs smoothly.

Here are a few ways you can help support your hormone balance:

- **Nutrition** – Eating a balanced diet rich in healthy fats, proteins, and essential vitamins and minerals can help your body produce and regulate hormones. For example, foods high in omega-3 fatty acids (like fish, flaxseeds, and walnuts) support hormone production, while antioxidants (found in fruits and vegetables) help reduce inflammation that can disrupt hormone balance.

- **Exercise** – Regular physical activity helps regulate hormones like insulin and cortisol, keeping your energy levels stable and reducing stress. Weight-bearing exercises also support bone health by encouraging the production of hormones like testosterone and estrogen.

- **Sleep** – Your body repairs and regenerates itself during sleep, and this includes regulating hormone levels. A good night's sleep helps balance cortisol and melatonin, ensuring you wake up feeling refreshed.

- **Stress Management** – Chronic stress can wreak havoc on your hormones, particularly cortisol and adrenaline. Practices like meditation, deep breathing, and yoga can help reduce stress and support hormone balance.

- **Bioidentical Hormone Replacement Therapy (BHRT)** – For women who experience significant hormonal imbalances, particularly around menopause, BHRT can offer a way to restore balance. Bioidentical hormones are identical in structure to the hormones your body naturally produces, making them a more natural option for hormone replacement.

Why Understanding Hormones Is Empowering

Knowledge is power, especially when it comes to your hormones. Many women go through life feeling like they have no control over their bodies, especially as they age. They may think that feeling tired, moody, or gaining weight is just a part of getting older.

But it does not have to be that way.

By understanding your hormones and how they affect your body, you can take steps to maintain balance and improve your quality of life at any age. Whether it is through lifestyle changes, natural supplements, or medical therapies like BHRT, there are many ways to support your hormonal health.

Hormones may be small, but they are mighty. They control some of the most critical functions in your body, and when they are balanced, they can help you feel younger, more energetic, and more vibrant.

In the next chapter, we will explore how your hormones change during your reproductive years and how to navigate those changes with confidence. From puberty to pregnancy and beyond, understanding your hormones is key to feeling your best.

Summary: Hormones 101 – What Are They and Why Do They Matter?

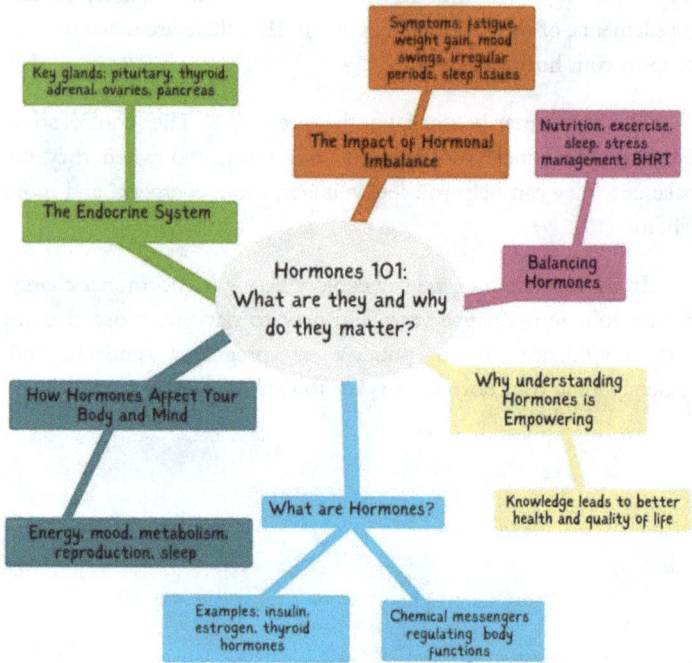

Symptoms: fatigue, weight gain, mood swings, irregular periods, sleep issues

Key glands: pituitary, thyroid, adrenal, ovaries, pancreas

The Impact of Hormonal Imbalance

Nutrition, excercise, sleep, stress management, BHRT

The Endocrine System

Hormones 101: What are they and why do they matter?

Balancing Hormones

How Hormones Affect Your Body and Mind

Why understanding Hormones is Empowering

Energy, mood, metabolism, reproduction, sleep

What are Hormones?

Knowledge leads to better health and quality of life

Examples: insulin, estrogen, thyroid hormones

Chemical messengers regulating body functions

Chapter 2
Puberty to Pregnancy
– Hormones in Your
Reproductive Years

The reproductive years in a woman's life are full of changes, transitions, and challenges, all driven by the powerful force of hormones. From the onset of puberty to the complexities of pregnancy, hormones play a central role in shaping your physical and emotional well-being. Understanding how your hormones work during these key stages can empower you to navigate them with greater ease and confidence.

In the following pages, we will explore how hormones influence your body from puberty through pregnancy, including common conditions like polycystic ovary syndrome (PCOS), endometriosis, and fertility challenges.

Puberty: The Hormonal Kick-Start

Puberty is the first major hormonal milestone in a woman's life. It usually begins between the ages of 8 and 13, as the body starts producing higher levels of sex hormones—primarily **estrogen** and **progesterone**—in preparation for reproduction. These hormones cause physical changes like breast development, pubic hair growth, and the start of menstruation.

What Happens During Puberty?

Puberty can feel like a whirlwind because so many changes are happening at once. Here is a breakdown of the primary hormonal shifts:

- **Estrogen Surge**: Estrogen is the primary female sex hormone and plays a considerable role in puberty. It causes breast development, the growth of the uterus, and the start of menstrual cycles. Estrogen also affects mood and brain development, which is why many girls experience emotional ups and downs during this time.

- **Progesterone's Role**: While estrogen is in the spotlight, **progesterone** works behind the scenes, preparing your body for pregnancy and regulating the menstrual cycle. It helps thicken the lining of the uterus, creating a nurturing environment for a fertilised egg.

- **Follicle-Stimulating Hormone (FSH) and Luteinising Hormone (LH)**: These hormones, produced by the pituitary gland, trigger the ovaries to release eggs. FSH stimulates the growth of ovarian follicles (where eggs are housed), and LH causes ovulation—the release of an egg from the ovary.

For many young women, puberty can bring irregular periods, mood swings, acne, and growing pains. These changes are all part of the body's hormonal adjustment to its new reproductive capabilities.

Menstruation: The Monthly Cycle

Once puberty is fully underway, most girls begin to experience regular menstrual cycles. This monthly cycle is orchestrated by a complex interplay of hormones that prepare the body for pregnancy.

Here is a simple breakdown of how it works:

1. **The Follicular Phase** (Day 1-14): The cycle begins with the first day of menstruation (Day 1), when the uterus sheds its lining. During this time, levels of **FSH** rise, stimulating the ovaries to produce follicles. One of these follicles will mature into an egg.

2. **Ovulation** (Day 14): Midway through the cycle, a spike in **LH** triggers the release of the egg from the ovary. This is called

ovulation. The egg then travels down the fallopian tube, where it may be fertilised by sperm.

3. **The Luteal Phase** (Day 15-28): After ovulation, the empty follicle transforms into the **corpus luteum**, which produces **progesterone**. Progesterone helps thicken the uterine lining in case of pregnancy. If the egg is not fertilised, progesterone levels drop, and the cycle starts over with menstruation.

While the menstrual cycle is a sign of a healthy reproductive system, it can also be accompanied by PMS (premenstrual syndrome), cramps, and other symptoms caused by fluctuating hormone levels.

Common Hormonal Conditions in the Reproductive Years

While many women experience regular, symptom-free cycles, others may face hormonal imbalances that lead to conditions like **Polycystic Ovary Syndrome (PCOS)** or **Endometriosis**. These conditions can affect fertility, energy levels, and overall well-being.

Polycystic Ovary Syndrome (PCOS)

PCOS is one of the most common hormonal disorders in women of reproductive age. It occurs when the ovaries produce excess androgens (male hormones), which can interfere with normal ovulation.

Symptoms of PCOS include:

- Irregular periods or no periods at all

- Excess facial or body hair (hirsutism)

- Acne or oily skin

- Weight gain, particularly around the abdomen

- Difficulty getting pregnant

The exact cause of PCOS is still unknown, but it is thought to involve insulin resistance, which can lead to higher levels of androgens. This hormone imbalance disrupts the menstrual cycle and can affect fertility.

Managing PCOS often involves lifestyle changes, such as maintaining a healthy weight, regular exercise, and a balanced diet to help regulate insulin levels. Some women may also benefit from medications like birth control pills or metformin to manage symptoms and restore hormonal balance.

Endometriosis

Endometriosis occurs when tissue similar to the lining of the uterus grows outside the uterus, often on the ovaries, fallopian tubes, or other pelvic organs. This tissue responds to hormonal changes during the menstrual cycle, leading to inflammation, pain, and sometimes infertility.

Symptoms of endometriosis include:

- Severe menstrual cramps

- Pain during or after sex

- Heavy periods or spotting between periods

- Infertility

Endometriosis can be difficult to diagnose, as its symptoms are similar to those of other conditions. Treatment often includes pain management, hormone therapy to reduce estrogen levels (which fuel endometrial tissue growth), and sometimes surgery to remove endometrial tissue.

Fertility Challenges

Hormonal imbalances during the reproductive years can also lead to fertility challenges. Ovulation disorders, such as those caused by PCOS or thyroid dysfunction, are among the most common causes of infertility in women. Other factors, such as blocked fallopian tubes, low egg quality, or endometriosis, can also impact fertility.

While hormonal treatments like **Clomid** (which stimulates ovulation) or **IVF** (In Vitro Fertilisation) can help many women conceive, it is essential to understand how your hormones are functioning if you are facing fertility challenges. Regular monitoring of hormones like **FSH**, **LH**, **estrogen**, and **progesterone** can provide valuable insight into your reproductive health.

Pregnancy: The Ultimate Hormonal Balancing Act

Pregnancy is a time of profound hormonal change. During these nine months, your body produces higher levels of hormones to support the growing baby and prepare for childbirth.

Here is a look at some of the key hormones during pregnancy:

- **Human Chorionic Gonadotropin (hCG)**: This hormone is produced by the placenta shortly after the fertilised egg attaches to the uterine lining. It helps maintain the corpus luteum and supports early pregnancy.

- **Progesterone**: Progesterone levels soar during pregnancy, helping to thicken the uterine lining, prevent contractions, and support the growth of the placenta. It also relaxes the muscles in your uterus, preventing premature labour.

- **Estrogen**: Estrogen plays a crucial role in fetal development, regulating the growth of the baby's organs and the expansion of the uterus. It also increases blood flow to the uterus and breasts, preparing the body for breastfeeding.

- **Relaxin**: This hormone helps relax the ligaments in your pelvis, preparing your body for childbirth. It also plays a role in preventing preterm labour.

While pregnancy is a time of excitement, it can also bring challenges like **morning sickness**, **fatigue**, and **mood swings**, all of which are influenced by fluctuating hormone levels.

For most women, the body's hormonal balancing act during pregnancy goes smoothly. However, conditions like **gestational diabetes** (caused by insulin resistance during pregnancy) or **pre-eclampsia** (a serious condition involving high blood pressure) can arise, requiring careful medical management.

Case Study: Hormones and Fertility – Sarah's Story

Sarah was a 32-year-old woman who had been trying to conceive for over a year without success. She had regular periods but noticed they were becoming more irregular, with some months where her cycle stretched beyond 35 days. She also experienced severe PMS symptoms, including mood swings, bloating, and fatigue.

After consulting her doctor, Sarah was diagnosed with **PCOS**. Blood tests revealed elevated levels of androgens and insulin resistance, both common markers of the condition.

Sarah began a treatment plan that included lifestyle changes, such as following a low-glycemic diet to manage her insulin levels and incorporating regular exercise. Her doctor also prescribed **metformin** to help regulate her insulin resistance and a low-dose birth control pill to manage her hormone levels.

After several months of treatment, Sarah's cycles became more regular, and she began ovulating consistently. She eventually conceived and successfully carried a healthy pregnancy to term.

Sarah's story highlights the importance of understanding the role hormones play in fertility. By addressing the underlying hormonal imbalance, she was able to improve her chances of conception.

Hormonal Health in Your 20s and 30s: The Takeaway

Your reproductive years are marked by significant hormonal changes, and understanding how these changes affect your body can help you manage your health more effectively. Whether you are dealing with PCOS, endometriosis, or fertility challenges, taking control of your hormonal health is vital to living a full, balanced life.

Here are a few tips for supporting your hormones during these critical years:

1. **Eat a balanced diet** rich in healthy fats, lean proteins, and whole grains to support hormone production.

2. **Exercise regularly** to help regulate insulin and support reproductive health.

3. **Manage stress**, which can have a significant impact on hormonal balance, particularly cortisol and androgens.

4. **Monitor your menstrual cycle** and consult a healthcare provider if you notice irregularities or have trouble conceiving.

5. **Seek medical advice** if you are experiencing symptoms like painful periods, acne, or excessive hair growth, as these could be signs of a hormonal imbalance.

In the next chapter, we will dive into the hormonal changes that occur during **perimenopause and menopause**—a new phase in hormonal health that many women experience in their 40s and beyond. Understanding these changes can help you navigate this transition with greater confidence and well-being.

Navigating the Reproductive Years

Your reproductive years are defined by hormonal shifts that can affect every aspect of your health and well-being. By understanding how hormones influence your menstrual cycle, fertility, and pregnancy, you can make informed choices about your health and take proactive steps to maintain hormonal balance.

Here are a few key takeaways for supporting your hormones during these years:

- **Maintain a balanced diet** rich in healthy fats, lean proteins, and whole grains to support hormone production.

- **Exercise regularly**, as physical activity can help regulate insulin levels and support reproductive health.

- **Manage stress**, as chronic stress can lead to hormonal imbalances and impact fertility.

- **Consult with a healthcare provider** if you experience irregular periods, painful symptoms, or difficulty conceiving.

In the next chapter, we will dive into the hormonal changes that occur during **perimenopause and menopause**. Understanding these changes can help you navigate this transition with greater confidence and well-being.

Summary: Puberty to Pregnancy – Hormones in Your Reproductive Years

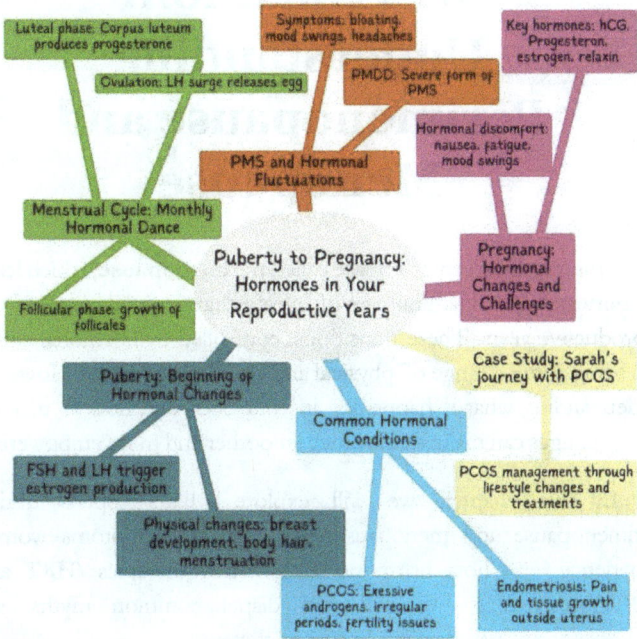

Luteal phase. Corpus luteum produces progesterone

Symptoms: bloating, mood swings, headaches

Key hormones: hCG, Progesteron, estrogen, relaxin

Ovulation: LH surge releases egg

PMDD: Severe form of PMS

Hormonal discomfort: nausea, fatigue, mood swings

PMS and Hormonal Fluctuations

Menstrual Cycle: Monthly Hormonal Dance

Puberty to Pregnancy: Hormones in Your Reproductive Years

Pregnancy: Hormonal Changes and Challenges

Follicular phase: growth of follicales

Case Study: Sarah's journey with PCOS

Puberty: Beginning of Hormonal Changes

Common Hormonal Conditions

PCOS management through lifestyle changes and treatments

FSH and LH trigger estrogen production

Physical changes: breast development, body hair, menstruation

PCOS: Exessive androgens, irregular periods, fertility issues

Endometriosis: Pain and tissue growth outside uterus

Chapter 3
The Transition – Understanding Perimenopause and Menopause

As women age, they enter a phase called **perimenopause**, which leads to **menopause**—a natural part of ageing that marks the end of the reproductive years. These transitions, controlled by hormonal shifts, can bring about a range of physical and emotional changes. However, understanding what is happening in your body and how to manage these changes can make this journey smoother and more empowering.

In this chapter, we will explore what happens during perimenopause and menopause, the common symptoms women experience, and how hormone replacement therapies (HRT and BHRT) can help. We will also dispel common myths and misconceptions surrounding hormone therapy.

Perimenopause: The Roller Coaster of Hormonal Changes

Think of **perimenopause** as the hormonal prelude to menopause. It can start as early as a woman's late 30s or early 40s, but the exact timing varies from person to person. During perimenopause, the ovaries gradually produce less **estrogen** and **progesterone**, the key hormones that regulate the menstrual cycle and many other bodily functions.

Think of your body as an orchestra, with hormones as the musicians playing in harmony. As perimenopause approaches, some musicians begin to miss rehearsals, play out of tune, or even leave the orchestra altogether. This disharmony creates the varied and often unpredictable symphony of symptoms women experience during this transition.

Symptoms of Perimenopause

Some women glide through perimenopause with few noticeable changes, while others experience a host of symptoms. The symptoms you experience are the result of hormonal fluctuations and can include:

- **Irregular periods**: Periods may become lighter, heavier, or more unpredictable as your hormone levels fluctuate.

- **Hot flushes and night sweats**: Sudden waves of heat that make you feel flushed and sweaty, often followed by chills.

- **Mood swings**: Just like during PMS, fluctuating hormone levels can cause irritability, anxiety, or sadness.

- **Sleep disturbances**: You may have trouble falling asleep or staying asleep, particularly if night sweats wake you up.

- **Weight gain**: Many women notice changes in body weight, especially around the abdomen, due to shifting hormone levels.

- **Brain fog**: Difficulty concentrating or remembering things can be frustrating and is often linked to hormonal shifts.

- **Decreased libido**: A drop in sexual desire is common during perimenopause, as hormone levels decrease.

Perimenopause can last anywhere from a few months to several years, culminating in menopause—the point at which you have gone 12 consecutive months without a period.

Menopause: The End of Menstruation

Menopause officially begins after a woman's final menstrual period. This means your ovaries are no longer releasing eggs, and your production of estrogen and progesterone has significantly decreased. For many women, menopause happens in their late 40s or early 50s, but just like perimenopause, the timing varies.

While menopause is a natural part of ageing, it is often viewed with a sense of dread due to the uncomfortable symptoms associated with it. However, menopause is simply a transition, and with the right approach, women can thrive during and after this stage of life.

Symptoms of Menopause

Many of the symptoms experienced during perimenopause will continue into menopause, including:

- **Hot flushes and night sweats:** These are often the hallmark symptoms of menopause and can last for several years.

- **Vaginal dryness:** As estrogen levels drop, vaginal tissue can become thinner and less lubricated, leading to discomfort during intercourse.

- **Mood changes:** Depression, anxiety, and mood swings can persist, particularly if sleep is being disrupted.

- **Bone loss:** Estrogen plays a crucial role in maintaining bone density. Without enough estrogen, women are at increased risk for osteoporosis, a condition that weakens the bones.

- **Heart health:** Menopause can increase the risk of heart disease, as estrogen has a protective effect on the cardiovascular system.

Just as the transition into menopause is gradual, the symptoms can be long-lasting. Some women experience these symptoms for only a few years, while others may deal with them for a decade or more.

Hormone Replacement Therapy (HRT) and Bioidentical Hormone Replacement Therapy (BHRT)

One of the most effective ways to manage the symptoms of perimenopause and menopause is through **Hormone Replacement Therapy (HRT)**. HRT works by replacing the hormones your body is no longer producing, helping to balance out the fluctuations that cause discomfort.

Traditional HRT vs. BHRT

- **Traditional HRT** uses synthetic hormones to replace estrogen and progesterone. These medications are designed to alleviate symptoms such as hot flushes, mood swings, and vaginal dryness, and reduce osteoporosis risk.

- **Bioidentical Hormone Replacement Therapy (BHRT)**, on the other hand, uses hormones that are chemically identical to the ones your body produces naturally. These hormones are often derived from plant sources and can be customised to meet an individual's specific needs.

Analogy: Think of HRT as putting oil in a car's engine when it is low—it helps everything run smoothly again. Traditional HRT is like using a generic oil that works for most cars, while BHRT is like using a specialised oil tailored to the exact specifications of your engine.

Benefits of Hormone Replacement Therapy

1. **Relief from Symptoms**: HRT and BHRT can effectively reduce the severity and frequency of hot flushes, night sweats, and mood swings.

2. **Improved Vaginal Health**: HRT can help maintain vaginal tissue health, improving lubrication and reducing discomfort during intercourse.

3. **Protection Against Bone Loss**: Estrogen replacement therapy is highly effective in preventing osteoporosis and reducing the risk of fractures.

4. **Heart Health**: Estrogen has a protective effect on the cardiovascular system, so replacing it may help reduce the risk of heart disease.

Myths About Hormone Therapy

There are several myths and misconceptions about hormone therapy, particularly when it comes to safety. Let us debunk some of the most common myths:

- **Myth 1: Hormone Therapy Causes Cancer** While there is some concern about the link between hormone therapy and certain types of cancer, research shows that the risks are often exaggerated. For women under 60 or within 10 years of menopause, the benefits of HRT often outweigh the risks, especially when it comes to protecting bone and heart health.

- **Myth 2: All Hormone Therapies Are the Same** Not all hormone therapies are created equal. BHRT, for example, is often preferred by women because it uses hormones that are identical to the ones naturally produced by the body. This can result in fewer side effects and a more customised approach to treatment.

- **Myth 3: Hormone Therapy is Only for Severe Symptoms** Even if your symptoms are mild, hormone therapy can help maintain overall health during and after menopause. Estrogen replacement can protect against bone loss and reduce the risk of heart disease, which may not be immediately noticeable but has long-term health benefits.

Is Hormone Therapy Right for You?

Hormone therapy is not a one-size-fits-all solution, and whether it is right for you depends on your individual health profile. It is important to work closely with your healthcare provider to discuss the potential benefits and risks of hormone therapy, especially if you have a history of certain health conditions like breast cancer or blood clots.

Non-Hormonal Options for Managing Symptoms

Not all women will choose hormone therapy, and that is perfectly okay. There are plenty of non-hormonal strategies for managing the symptoms of perimenopause and menopause:

- **Diet and Nutrition**: A diet rich in calcium, vitamin D, and omega-3 fatty acids can support bone and heart health. Reducing caffeine, alcohol, and spicy foods may help with Hot flushes and night sweats.

- **Exercise**: Regular physical activity helps maintain a healthy weight, reduces the risk of heart disease, and strengthens bones.

- **Stress Management**: Mindfulness practices like yoga, meditation, and deep breathing can help manage mood swings and reduce anxiety.

- **Herbal Supplements**: Some women find relief from symptoms using herbal supplements like **black cohosh, evening primrose oil**, or **red clover**, though it is important to discuss these with your healthcare provider before starting any new supplements.

Case Study: Jane's Perimenopause Journey

Jane, a 47-year-old marketing executive, began experiencing **hot flushes, night sweats**, and **mood swings** in her early 40s. Her once-regular menstrual cycle had become erratic, and she often found herself feeling irritable and exhausted. Jane's symptoms were impacting her work and personal life, leaving her feeling overwhelmed.

After discussing her options with her doctor, Jane decided to try **BHRT**, opting for a personalised approach that matched her body's natural hormones. Within a few weeks, she noticed a significant reduction in her hot flushes, her mood stabilised, and she was sleeping better. While she initially had concerns about hormone therapy, Jane was relieved to find a solution that improved her quality of life during perimenopause.

Jane's story is a reminder that perimenopause and menopause, while challenging, can be managed with the right approach. Whether through hormone therapy or lifestyle changes, women can find relief and thrive during this transition.

Navigating Menopause with Confidence

Perimenopause and menopause are natural phases of life, not something to fear or dread. Understanding the hormonal changes behind these transitions can help you make informed choices about your health, from managing symptoms to protecting your bones and heart. Whether you choose hormone therapy or natural approaches, the key is finding what works best for you.

In the next chapter, we will explore the benefits of **Bioidentical Hormone Replacement Therapy (BHRT)** in more detail and how it differs from traditional hormone therapy.

Summary: The Transition – Understanding Perimenopause and Menopause

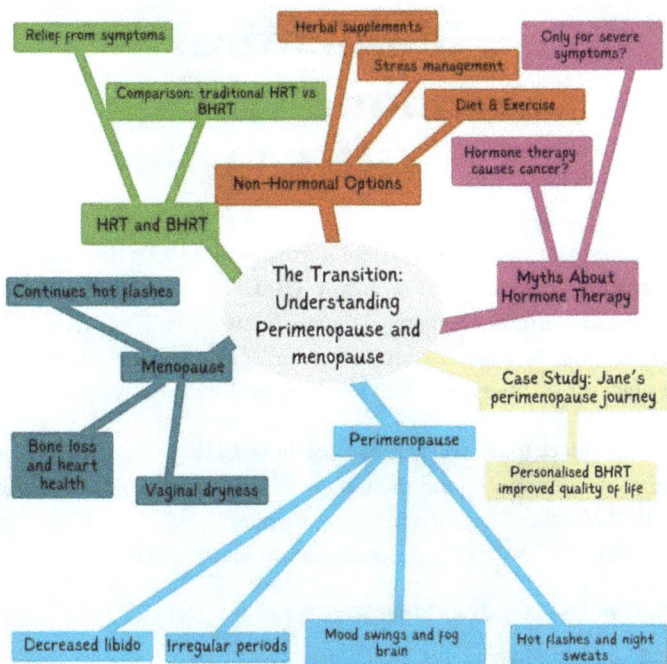

The Transition: Understanding Perimenopause and menopause

- Relief from symptoms
- Comparison: traditional HRT vs BHRT
- HRT and BHRT

- Herbal supplements
- Stress management
- Diet & Exercise
- Non-Hormonal Options

- Only for severe symptoms?
- Hormone therapy causes cancer?
- Myths About Hormone Therapy

- Continues hot flashes
- Menopause
- Bone loss and heart health
- Vaginal dryness

- Case Study: Jane's perimenopause journey
- Personalised BHRT improved quality of life

- Perimenopause
- Decreased libido
- Irregular periods
- Mood swings and fog brain
- Hot flashes and night sweats

Chapter 4
The Benefits of
Bioidentical
Hormone Therapy
(BHRT)

In recent years, many women have started to hear about **Bioidentical Hormone Replacement Therapy (BHRT)** as an alternative to traditional hormone therapy. You might wonder: What exactly is BHRT, and how is it different from the standard **Hormone Replacement Therapy (HRT)** offered by doctors for years?

In this chapter, we will explore how BHRT works, why it is becoming so popular, and the unique benefits it offers. We will also break down the differences between traditional HRT and BHRT so you can make informed choices about your hormonal health.

What is Bioidentical Hormone Therapy (BHRT)?

BHRT is a type of hormone therapy that uses hormones that are chemically identical to the ones produced naturally in your body. These bioidentical hormones can include **estrogen**, **progesterone**, **testosterone**, and **DHEA**, among others. BHRT is often used to treat symptoms of perimenopause, menopause, and other hormonal imbalances by restoring hormone levels to their optimal range.

Here is an easy analogy: Imagine your body is like a smartphone that is running low on battery. Hormones are like the power source that keeps everything functioning. When the power starts to drop, your phone—or body—begins to slow down and show signs of wear. BHRT acts like a custom-built charger that gives you exactly the power you need to get back to optimal functioning. Unlike traditional HRT, which uses synthetic hormones, BHRT gives your body a natural and precise "power boost."

How BHRT Differs from Traditional HRT

The primary difference between BHRT and traditional HRT lies in the hormones used:

- **Traditional HRT**: This therapy uses synthetic hormones or those derived from animal sources. One common example is **conjugated equine estrogen** (CEE), derived from the urine of pregnant horses, which has been used for many years in standard hormone therapies.

- **BHRT**: These hormones are chemically identical to those your body produces naturally. They are often made from plant sources, such as **soybeans** and **wild yams**, but they are modified in the lab to have the same molecular structure as human hormones. This "bioidentical" structure allows your body to recognise and use the hormones more efficiently.

Analogy: If traditional HRT is like receiving a general charger that might not perfectly fit your phone's port, BHRT is like having a custom charger made specifically for your device, ensuring it connects properly and works smoothly.

Personalisation with BHRT

Another critical advantage of BHRT is that it can be **personalised**. Doctors often work with **compounding pharmacies** to create custom hormone dosages based on each patient's unique needs. This means you get the exact hormones, in the precise amounts, that your body requires to function optimally.

The Benefits of BHRT

Now that we understand what BHRT is and how it works, let us dive into the specific benefits it offers.

1. Fewer Side Effects and Better Tolerance

One of the biggest advantages of BHRT is that, because the hormones are identical to those your body naturally produces, they tend to be better tolerated. Many women report fewer side effects compared to traditional HRT. This is because your body recognises the bioidentical hormones and can process them more easily.

Analogy: Think of it like switching from a generic, one-size-fits-all skincare product to one that is custom-made for your skin type. The custom product is likely to cause fewer reactions and work more effectively because it is designed to suit your unique needs.

Case Study: Sarah's Experience with BHRT

Sarah, a 52-year-old teacher, had been struggling with menopause symptoms for two years. She experienced **hot flushes**, **night sweats**, **mood swings**, and **brain fog**. Traditional HRT helped reduce some of her symptoms, but she disliked the side effects, including weight gain and bloating.

After switching to BHRT, Sarah noticed a significant improvement. Her hot flushes and night sweats decreased, her mood stabilised, and she felt mentally sharper. Best of all, the side effects she experienced on traditional HRT disappeared. Sarah's case is an example of how BHRT can offer a more tailored approach, resulting in better symptom control with fewer unwanted effects.

2. Customised Dosages for Your Unique Needs

With BHRT, your healthcare provider can prescribe dosages specifically tailored to your hormonal levels. This customisation allows for more precise hormone balancing, reducing the risk of side effects that often come with standard, one-size-fits-all HRT dosages.

Analogy: Imagine going to a tailor for a custom-fitted outfit versus buying something off the rack. The custom outfit fits perfectly, while the store-bought one might be too tight in some places or too loose in others. BHRT offers that same custom fit for your hormones.

3. Improved Quality of Life

Many women who switch to BHRT report a significant improvement in their overall quality of life. By restoring hormonal balance, BHRT can help reduce common menopause symptoms like **fatigue**, **irritability**, **hot flushes**, and **insomnia**.

Cognitive Function: BHRT can also help improve brain function. Estrogen, in particular, has a protective effect on the brain, supporting memory and cognitive function. Women on BHRT often report feeling sharper and more focused, with fewer episodes of brain fog.

Mood and Emotional Health: Hormonal imbalances can have a huge impact on mood, leading to **anxiety**, **depression**, and **irritability**. By replenishing hormones, BHRT can help stabilise mood and improve emotional well-being.

Bone Health: Estrogen plays a critical role in maintaining bone density. Without enough estrogen, women are at increased risk for **osteoporosis**. BHRT helps protect bone health by maintaining estrogen levels, reducing the risk of fractures and bone loss.

Heart Health: Hormones like estrogen also have a protective effect on the cardiovascular system, reducing the risk of heart disease. BHRT can help maintain heart health, particularly for women in the years following menopause.

Case Study: Emma's Journey with BHRT

Emma, a 49-year-old accountant, had been feeling run down for years. She was constantly tired, struggling to focus, and had lost her usual zest for life. Her symptoms, including **brain fog**, **weight gain**, and **joint pain**, had gradually worsened as she entered menopause. After a detailed consultation, Emma's doctor prescribed a custom blend of BHRT to address her hormonal deficiencies. Within three months, Emma felt like a new person. Her energy levels returned, her brain fog cleared, and she was back to enjoying her daily walks. Emma's story is a testament to how BHRT can transform the way women feel as they navigate menopause.

4. Fewer Health Risks Compared to Traditional HRT

Another important benefit of BHRT is that it is often associated with fewer health risks compared to traditional HRT, particularly when it comes to long-term use. Some studies suggest that BHRT, particularly **bioidentical progesterone**, may have a lower risk of certain conditions like **breast cancer** compared to synthetic hormones.

Analogy: It is like using a cleaner, more natural ingredient in your diet or skincare routine. Bioidentical hormones are thought to be processed by the body more smoothly, which could lead to fewer long-term risks.

Myths and Misconceptions about BHRT

Just like traditional HRT, BHRT is often misunderstood. Let us take a look at some of the common myths and misconceptions:

- **Myth 1: BHRT is not as well-researched as traditional HRT.** While it is true that bioidentical hormones have not been studied as extensively as synthetic hormones, there is growing research to support the safety and effectiveness of BHRT. Many women have used it successfully to manage their symptoms and improve their overall health.

- **Myth 2: BHRT is only for women in menopause.** While BHRT is commonly used for menopause symptoms, it can also be used to treat other hormonal imbalances, including **perimenopause, adrenal fatigue**, and **thyroid issues**. BHRT is beneficial for women in different stages of life, from their 30s onward.

- **Myth 3: BHRT is risk-free.** Although BHRT has many benefits, it is important to remember that it is still hormone therapy and should be monitored closely by a healthcare provider. Like any medical treatment, BHRT should be customised to the individual, and its effects should be regularly evaluated.

Is BHRT Right for You?

Whether you are just beginning to experience the symptoms of **perimenopause** or you are deep into **menopause**, BHRT might be the right choice for you if:

- You are looking for a **natural** approach to hormone therapy.
- You have tried traditional HRT but experienced **unpleasant side effects**.
- You want a **personalised** hormone treatment plan tailored to your specific needs.

Working with a Healthcare Provider

It is important to work with a healthcare provider who is experienced in prescribing BHRT. They will take the time to understand your symptoms, run the necessary tests, and create a custom treatment plan that fits your needs.

BHRT can be delivered in a variety of forms, including **creams, lozenges, pills**, or **patches**, depending on what works best for your lifestyle and body. Your healthcare provider will guide you through the process, ensuring your dosage is optimised and adjusted as needed.

Case Study: Laura's Customised BHRT Treatment

Laura, a 56-year-old artist, had been suffering from a lack of energy and a deep sense of emotional flatness. Her healthcare provider ran comprehensive hormone tests and discovered low levels of **progesterone, estrogen**, and **testosterone**. Based on her unique profile, Laura's doctor created a custom BHRT plan using a combination of **progesterone cream, estradiol lozenges**, and a low dose of **testosterone cream**. Within weeks, Laura felt more balanced, had more energy, and even noticed an improvement in her creativity and artistic work.

Conclusion: The Benefits of BHRT for Lifelong Vitality

BHRT offers a natural, personalised, and potentially safer alternative to traditional hormone therapies. By restoring your body's natural hormone balance, BHRT can improve your quality of life, protect your long-term health, and help you navigate hormonal changes with greater ease and confidence.

As we move forward in the book, we will continue to explore how hormones influence every aspect of your health and how you can take control of your hormonal health for lifelong vitality. In the next chapter, we will look at how hormones play a role in ageing, vitality, and overall health beyond menopause.

Summary: The Benefits of Bioidentical Hormone Therapy (BHRT)

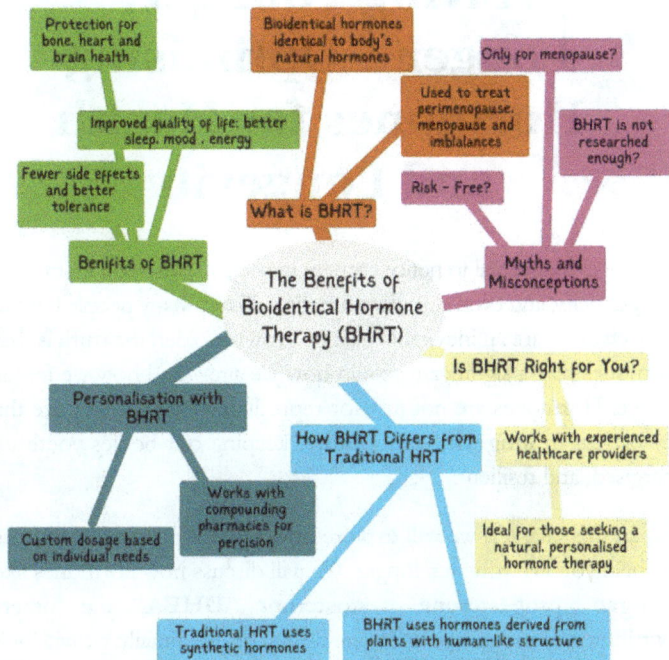

- Protection for bone, heart and brain health
- Bioidentical hormones identical to body's natural hormones
- Only for menopause?
- Improved quality of life: better sleep, mood, energy
- Used to treat perimenopause, menopause and imbalances
- BHRT is not researched enough?
- Fewer side effects and better tolerance
- Risk – Free?
- What is BHRT?
- Benifits of BHRT
- Myths and Misconceptions
- The Benefits of Bioidentical Hormone Therapy (BHRT)
- Is BHRT Right for You?
- Personalisation with BHRT
- How BHRT Differs from Traditional HRT
- Works with experienced healthcare providers
- Works with compounding pharmacies for percision
- Custom dosage based on individual needs
- Ideal for those seeking a natural, personalised hormone therapy
- Traditional HRT uses synthetic hormones
- BHRT uses hormones derived from plants with human-like structure

Chapter 5
Living Younger, Longer – Optimising Hormones for Health and Longevity

As we age, it is natural to notice changes in energy levels, muscle strength, skin elasticity, and even cognitive function. While many people believe these changes are an inevitable part of growing older, the truth is that hormones play a significant role in how we age—and how we feel as we age. Hormones are not just for reproductive health; they are the key players in **longevity** and **vitality**, keeping our bodies youthful, energised, and resilient.

In this chapter, we will explore how optimising your hormones can help you live younger, longer. We will discuss how hormones like **estrogen**, **progesterone**, **testosterone**, **DHEA**, and others contribute to various aspects of ageing and health. Finally, we will look at strategies for using hormone therapy to maintain strength, cognitive function, and overall well-being as you grow older.

How Hormones Influence Ageing

Hormones are often thought of as the messengers that control puberty, menstruation, and reproduction, but they do so much more. They regulate metabolism, energy production, immune function, and even the repair of tissues. As we age, the natural decline in hormone levels—especially in women during **perimenopause** and **menopause**—can lead to many of the signs of ageing we see and feel, such as fatigue, muscle loss, and memory problems.

To better understand how hormones affect ageing, imagine your body as a well-maintained car engine. When you are younger, the engine runs smoothly, delivering power and efficiency. However, over time, the engine's vital fluids (in this case, hormones) start to deplete. If you do not regularly refill and maintain those fluids, the engine starts to stutter, losing power, and eventually breaks down. Hormones are like the oil and fuel that keep your body's engine running efficiently. Optimising hormone levels as you age is like giving your engine the maintenance it needs to run smoothly for years to come.

1. Estrogen and Ageing

Estrogen is not just a reproductive hormone. It plays a critical role in maintaining **bone health**, **skin elasticity**, **heart health**, and **brain function**. After menopause, when estrogen levels drop, women are more vulnerable to conditions like **osteoporosis**, **heart disease**, and **cognitive decline**. The decline in estrogen can also contribute to dry skin, wrinkles, and loss of skin elasticity.

Optimising estrogen levels can help protect against these ageing-related conditions, keeping your bones strong, your skin youthful, and your brain sharp. In fact, studies have shown that estrogen replacement therapy can reduce the risk of **Alzheimer's disease** and **dementia** in women, which highlights the hormone's protective effects on the brain.

2. Progesterone's Role in Healthy Ageing

Progesterone works in tandem with estrogen, ensuring that the body stays in balance. It has a calming, **anti-inflammatory** effect on the body, which is particularly important as we age. Chronic inflammation is linked to many age-related diseases, including **arthritis**, **heart disease**, and **cognitive decline**.

In addition to its anti-inflammatory properties, progesterone helps maintain bone density and promote better sleep. As we age, **sleep quality** often diminishes, leading to increased fatigue and cognitive issues. By optimising progesterone levels, you can enjoy better sleep, lower stress levels, and reduced inflammation—factors that are crucial for staying young and healthy.

Case Study: Emma's Journey to Better Sleep and Health with Progesterone

Emma, a 55-year-old grandmother, had been struggling with **insomnia** and **joint pain** for years. Her lack of sleep made her feel tired and sluggish during the day, and her joint pain limited her ability to stay active. After her doctor discovered her **low progesterone levels**, she began **bioidentical progesterone therapy**. Within a few weeks, Emma noticed a significant improvement in her sleep quality, which had a ripple effect on her energy levels, mood, and overall sense of well-being. Her joint pain also lessened, allowing her to return to her favourite activities, like gardening and yoga.

Emma's story shows how progesterone not only improves **sleep** but also contributes to overall vitality as we age.

3. Testosterone and Muscle Health

When people think of testosterone, they often associate it with men, but testosterone is essential for women's health as well. Testosterone plays a key role in maintaining **muscle mass**, **bone strength**, **energy levels**, and **libido**. As women age, testosterone levels naturally decline, leading to **muscle loss**, **fatigue**, and **reduced sexual desire**.

Maintaining optimal testosterone levels can help prevent **sarcopenia** (age-related muscle loss) and keep your muscles strong and healthy. It also supports metabolism, helping to prevent the weight gain that often comes with age.

Analogy: Think of testosterone as the scaffolding that supports the building that is your body. When the scaffolding weakens, the entire structure starts to sag. By replenishing testosterone, you reinforce that scaffolding, keeping your body strong and upright.

Case Study: Lisa's Muscle Strength Journey with Testosterone

Lisa, a 49-year-old fitness instructor, noticed that despite regular exercise, she was losing muscle mass and strength. She felt constantly tired and found it harder to recover after her workouts. A blood test revealed that her **testosterone levels were low**. After starting **bioidentical testosterone therapy**, Lisa's strength returned, her energy levels increased, and she was able to continue teaching her fitness classes with the same vigour as she had in her younger years. Lisa's story shows how testosterone can be the key to maintaining strength and vitality as we age.

4. DHEA and Longevity

DHEA (Dehydroepiandrosterone) is often referred to as the "longevity hormone" because of its wide-reaching benefits in promoting health and vitality. DHEA is a precursor to other hormones like testosterone and estrogen, and it plays a crucial role in **immune function, energy levels**, and **cognitive health**.

As we age, DHEA levels decline, which can lead to **fatigue, low mood**, and even a weakened immune system. Optimising DHEA levels can help enhance **mental clarity, reduce stress**, and boost the immune system—key factors in staying healthy and vibrant as we grow older.

5. Pregnenolone: The "Mother Hormone"

Pregnenolone is another crucial hormone that acts as a precursor to many others, including **progesterone, estrogen**, and **testosterone**. It is sometimes called the **"mother hormone"** because it serves as the building block for a wide range of essential hormones.

Pregnenolone helps with **memory, cognitive function**, and **mood** regulation. As we age, declining pregnenolone levels can lead to **memory lapses, foggy thinking**, and **low mood**. By optimising pregnenolone, you can support brain health, improve memory, and reduce symptoms of **anxiety** and **depression** that often accompany ageing.

6. Cortisol: The Stress Hormone and Its Impact on Ageing

Cortisol, commonly known as the **stress hormone**, is essential for helping your body manage stress. However, chronically high cortisol levels can accelerate the ageing process, leading to **inflammation**, **weight gain**, **sleep disturbances**, and even **cognitive decline**.

It is important to maintain balanced cortisol levels through lifestyle measures like **stress management**, **adequate sleep**, and, when necessary, hormone optimisation. Reducing excess cortisol can protect your body from the damaging effects of chronic stress and promote **healthy ageing**.

Strategies for Optimising Hormones for Longevity

Now that we've explored the role of various hormones in ageing, let us look at some practical strategies for optimising your hormone levels to promote long-term health and vitality.

1. Hormone Testing and Monitoring

The first step in optimising your hormones is getting them tested by a healthcare provider. Hormone testing can reveal imbalances and deficiencies that may be contributing to your symptoms. Regular monitoring ensures that your hormone levels remain balanced over time, and any necessary adjustments to therapy can be made.

2. Bioidentical Hormone Therapy (BHRT)

BHRT offers a natural, personalised approach to hormone therapy, using hormones that are chemically identical to those your body produces. As we've discussed, BHRT can help restore hormone balance, protect against age-related diseases, and improve overall well-being.

3. Nutrition for Hormone Health

Certain foods can support healthy hormone levels, including:

- **Healthy fats** (like avocados, nuts, and olive oil) to support pregnenolone and DHEA production.

- **Cruciferous vegetables** (like broccoli and kale) to help metabolise excess estrogen.

- **Lean proteins** to support muscle health and testosterone production.

4. Exercise and Hormonal Balance

Strength training and **resistance exercises** are particularly effective for boosting testosterone and maintaining muscle mass. Regular **cardiovascular exercise** can help balance cortisol and improve heart health.

5. Stress Management

Because cortisol plays such a significant role in ageing, it is essential to manage chronic stress. Practices like **meditation, yoga,** and **deep breathing exercises** can help reduce cortisol levels and promote a sense of calm.

6. Sleep Optimisation

Quality sleep is crucial for hormone production and overall health. Aim for 7-9 hours of sleep per night and create a sleep-friendly environment by reducing light, noise, and stress before bedtime.

Conclusion: Living Younger, Longer with Hormonal Health

Optimising your hormone levels can be the key to living younger, longer. By maintaining balanced hormones, you can protect your bones, muscles, brain, and heart—ensuring a healthier, more vibrant life as you age. As we move forward, remember that ageing does not have to mean a decline in vitality. With the right tools and knowledge, you can keep your body functioning at its best, well into your golden years.

In the next chapter, we will explore how **nutrition, exercise**, and **lifestyle** can support your hormonal health naturally, further enhancing your well-being and longevity.

Summary: Living Younger, Longer – Optimising Hormones for Health and Longevity

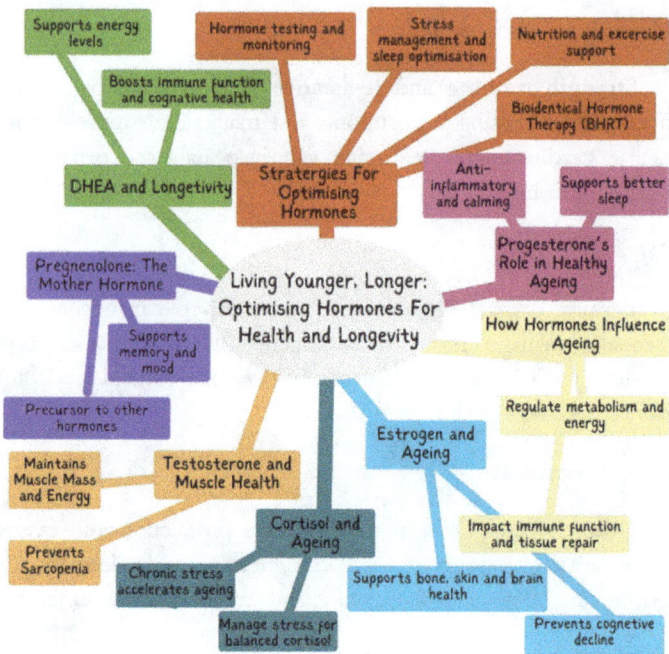

Living Younger, Longer: Optimising Hormones For Health and Longevity

- Stratergies For Optimising Hormones
  - Supports energy levels
  - Boosts immune function and cognative health
  - DHEA and Longetivity
  - Hormone testing and monitoring
  - Stress management and sleep optimisation
  - Nutrition and excercise support
  - Bioidentical Hormone Therapy (BHRT)
  - Anti-inflammatory and calming
  - Supports better sleep
  - Progesterone's Role in Healthy Ageing

- Pregnenolone: The Mother Hormone
  - Supports memory and mood
  - Precursor to other hormones

- How Hormones Influence Ageing
  - Regulate metabolism and energy
  - Impact immune function and tissue repair

- Testosterone and Muscle Health
  - Maintains Muscle Mass and Energy
  - Prevents Sarcopenia

- Cortisol and Ageing
  - Chronic stress accelerates ageing
  - Manage stress for balanced cortisol

- Estrogen and Ageing
  - Supports bone, skin and brain health
  - Prevents cognitive decline

Chapter 6
Natural Hormone Balancers – Nutrition, Exercise, and Stress Management

Hormone health is not just about what is happening inside your body—it is also heavily influenced by your daily choices, including the food you eat, the way you move, and how you manage stress. In this chapter, we will dive into natural ways to balance your hormones through nutrition, exercise, and stress management.

Consider your hormones as a team of skilled athletes working together to win a championship game. Each athlete plays a crucial role, and their coordinated efforts contribute to overall success. When one athlete is off their game – perhaps due to an injury or lack of training (representing a hormonal imbalance) – the entire team's performance is compromised. But with the right coaching and support (lifestyle adjustments), that athlete can regain their strength and the team can get back on track to victory.

The Role of Nutrition in Balancing Hormones

What you eat directly impacts how your hormones function. A balanced, nutrient-dense diet can help your body produce and regulate hormones. In contrast, a diet high in processed foods, sugars, and unhealthy fats can throw your hormones off balance. Let us look at how specific foods can support hormone health.

1. Healthy Fats for Hormone Production

Healthy fats are the building blocks of hormones. Without enough fat in your diet, your body can not produce the essential hormones like estrogen, progesterone, and testosterone that keep your body running smoothly.

Think of healthy fats as the fuel that powers your hormonal engine. Just as a car can not run without fuel, your body can not produce the necessary hormones without a steady supply of good fats. Include **avocados**, **nuts**, **seeds**, **olive oil**, and **fatty fish** like salmon in your diet to support hormone production.

2. Cruciferous Vegetables for Estrogen Balance

Cruciferous vegetables like **broccoli**, **kale**, and **Brussels sprouts** contain compounds that help your body metabolise and excrete excess estrogen. This is especially important for women, as an excess of estrogen relative to progesterone can lead to a condition known as **estrogen dominance**, which may cause symptoms like **weight gain**, **mood swings**, and **irregular periods**.

Think of cruciferous vegetables as your body's natural detoxifiers, helping to sweep out excess estrogen and keep your hormonal balance in check.

3. Protein for Muscle and Metabolism

Protein is essential for maintaining muscle mass, which is crucial for **testosterone** and **growth hormone** production. Without enough protein, your body may break down muscle tissue, which can lead to fatigue, weight gain, and slower metabolism.

Include lean proteins like **chicken**, **turkey**, **eggs** and **plant-based proteins** such as **lentils** and **chickpeas** in your diet. Protein is also necessary for keeping you full and satisfied, reducing cravings that can lead to overeating.

4. Fibre for Hormone Detoxification

Fibre helps regulate blood sugar levels and aids in hormone detoxification. It also supports gut health, which is closely linked to hormone production and balance. A healthy gut ensures that hormones like **insulin** and **cortisol** stay balanced, reducing the risk of **insulin resistance** and stress-related hormone imbalances.

Make sure to include plenty of fibre-rich foods like **whole grains**, **vegetables**, **fruits**, and **legumes** in your daily diet.

5. Avoiding Processed Sugars and Refined Carbohydrates

Processed sugars and refined carbohydrates cause spikes in blood sugar levels, leading to an overproduction of **insulin**. High insulin levels can disrupt hormone balance and contribute to conditions like **polycystic ovary syndrome (PCOS)**, **weight gain**, and **fatigue**.

By avoiding sugary snacks, sodas, and white bread, you can keep your blood sugar stable and prevent unnecessary strain on your hormone system.

Exercise and Hormone Balance

Exercise is another powerful tool for keeping your hormones in check. It does not just help you maintain a healthy weight—it also affects hormone levels, helping to reduce stress hormones like **cortisol** and boosting the production of **endorphins**, **testosterone**, and **growth hormone**.

1. Strength Training for Testosterone and Growth Hormone

Strength training, such as lifting weights or doing bodyweight exercises, is one of the best ways to boost **testosterone** and **growth hormone** production. These hormones are essential for building and maintaining muscle, as well as supporting metabolism and energy levels.

Imagine strength training as the conductor of your hormonal orchestra. When you lift weights, you are directing your body to produce the hormones that will help you feel stronger, more energised, and more capable of handling life's challenges.

2. Cardiovascular Exercise for Insulin Sensitivity and Heart Health

Cardiovascular exercise, such as walking, running, or cycling, helps improve **insulin sensitivity** and supports **heart health**. By doing regular cardio, you can lower your risk of **insulin resistance**, which is linked to conditions like **diabetes** and **obesity**.

Even moderate cardio exercises, such as brisk walking for 30 minutes a day, can make a big difference in keeping your insulin and other hormones in balance.

3. Yoga and Pilates for Stress Reduction and Cortisol Control

Yoga and **Pilates** are not only great for flexibility and core strength but also for reducing stress and lowering **cortisol** levels. Cortisol is a hormone that spikes in response to stress. While cortisol is helpful in short bursts, chronic stress and high cortisol levels can disrupt hormone balance, leading to **weight gain**, **fatigue**, and **anxiety**.

By practising yoga or Pilates regularly, you can lower your cortisol levels, improve your mood, and enhance overall hormonal balance.

Case Study: Maria's Transformation Through Exercise

Maria, a 45-year-old mother of two, was feeling sluggish and had gained weight over the past few years. She found it difficult to balance her busy lifestyle with self-care and rarely made time for exercise. After learning about the connection between strength training and hormone health, Maria decided to start working out with weights twice a week. She also added a daily 30-minute walk to her routine.

Within a few months, Maria noticed a significant improvement in her energy levels, mood, and overall sense of well-being. Her weight began to normalise, and she felt more in control of her body. The strength training helped her feel stronger and more confident, while the daily walks reduced her stress and anxiety.

Maria's story shows how regular exercise can be a game-changer for hormonal balance and overall health.

Stress Management and Hormone Health

Chronic stress is one of the biggest disruptors of hormonal balance. When you are stressed, your body produces excess **cortisol**, which can lead to a cascade of hormonal imbalances. High cortisol levels can deplete **progesterone**, elevate **insulin**, and even reduce **thyroid hormone** levels—all of which can contribute to weight gain, fatigue, and mood disorders.

1. Mindfulness and Meditation for Cortisol Control

Mindfulness and **meditation** are two of the most effective ways to manage stress and lower cortisol levels. These practices help calm the mind and body, promoting relaxation and reducing the fight-or-flight response that triggers cortisol production.

Think of mindfulness as hitting the pause button on your stress response. It allows your body to reset and brings you back to a state of calm, helping to keep cortisol levels in check.

2. Deep Breathing and Relaxation Techniques

Deep breathing exercises, such as **diaphragmatic breathing** or **box breathing**, can quickly reduce cortisol levels and promote a sense of calm. These techniques are easy to practise anywhere, whether you are at home, in the office, or on the go.

3. Quality Sleep for Hormonal Balance

Sleep is one of the most underrated factors in hormone health. Without enough sleep, your body can not properly regulate hormones like **cortisol, insulin, leptin,** and **ghrelin** (which control hunger and satiety). Poor sleep is linked to **weight gain, fatigue,** and **mood disorders**.

Aim for 7-9 hours of quality sleep each night. Creating a **sleep-friendly environment**, such as reducing light and noise, avoiding screens before bed, and maintaining a regular sleep schedule, can make a big difference in your hormonal health.

Case Study: Sophie's Stress Reduction Journey

Sophie, a 38-year-old entrepreneur, was constantly stressed from managing her business and raising two children. Her stress levels were through the roof, and she was starting to experience **weight gain**, **insomnia**, and **mood swings**. A hormone test revealed that Sophie's **cortisol levels were high**, which was likely contributing to her symptoms.

Sophie decided to make stress management a priority. She began practising **mindfulness meditation** for 10 minutes each morning and introduced **deep breathing exercises** before bed. After a few weeks, Sophie noticed that her sleep improved, her mood stabilised, and she felt more in control of her emotions.

Sophie's case shows how managing stress through mindfulness and relaxation techniques can have a profound impact on hormone health.

Natural Supplements to Support Hormone Health

While a balanced diet, regular exercise, and stress management are the foundations of hormone health, certain natural supplements can also support your hormonal balance. Here are a few essential supplements that can help:

- **Magnesium**: Supports relaxation, sleep, and stress reduction. Found in leafy greens, nuts, and seeds.

- **Zinc**: Helps with testosterone production and immune function. Found in shellfish, meats, and legumes.

- **Vitamin D**: Plays a crucial role in hormone production and immune health. Best sourced from sunlight but also found in fatty fish and fortified foods.

- **Ashwagandha**: An adaptogen that helps lower cortisol and manage stress.

- **Omega-3 Fatty Acids**: Supports hormone balance, brain health, and inflammation reduction. Found in fish like salmon and flaxseeds.

Conclusion: A Holistic Approach to Hormone Health

Maintaining balanced hormones naturally requires a holistic approach. By focusing on nutrition, exercise, stress management, and natural supplements, you can support your body's natural hormone production and create a foundation for long-term health and vitality.

In the next chapter, we will discuss how hormone changes affect your body through every decade of life—from your 20s to your 60s and beyond. By understanding these changes, you can tailor your lifestyle choices to support your hormonal health at every stage.

Summary: Natural Hormone Balancers – Nutrition, Exercise, and Stress Management

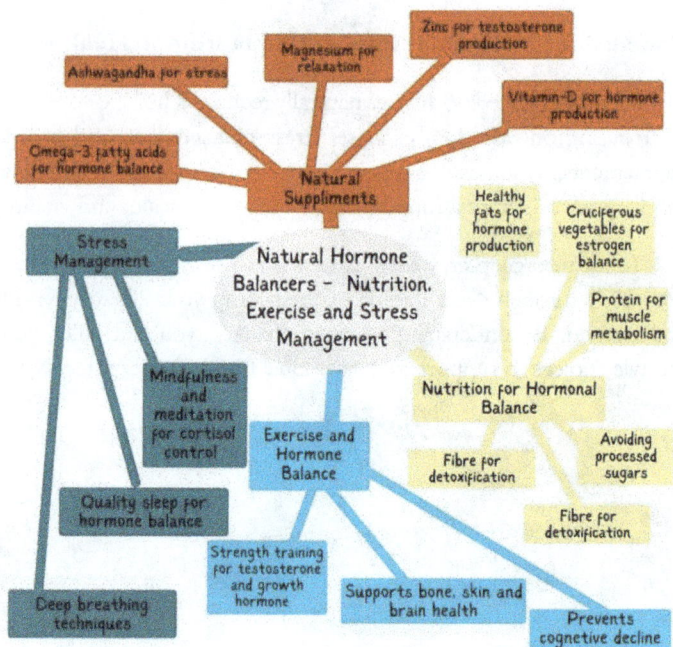

Natural Hormone Balancers – Nutrition, Exercise and Stress Management

Natural Suppliments
- Ashwagandha for stress
- Magnesium for relaxation
- Zinc for testosterone production
- Vitamin-D for hormone production
- Omega-3 fatty acids for hormone balance

Stress Management
- Mindfulness and meditation for cortisol control
- Quality sleep for hormone balance
- Deep breathing techniques

Exercise and Hormone Balance
- Strength training for testosterone and growth hormone
- Supports bone, skin and brain health
- Prevents cognetive decline

Nutrition for Hormonal Balance
- Healthy fats for hormone production
- Cruciferous vegetables for estrogen balance
- Protein for muscle metabolism
- Fibre for detoxification
- Avoiding processed sugars
- Fibre for detoxification

Chapter 7
Navigating Hormonal Changes Through Every Decade

Hormones are your body's master messengers. These chemical signals influence everything from your mood and energy levels to your reproductive health, skin quality, and even your metabolism. Understanding how hormones change as you age is crucial for maintaining health and well-being through every phase of life. This chapter takes a deeper look at how hormonal shifts occur in each decade of a woman's life, why they matter, and what steps you can take to optimise hormonal balance through every stage.

Your 20s: The Reproductive Prime

In your 20s, your hormones are running at peak performance. This is often the decade where women feel the most energetic, fertile, and physically resilient. However, that does not mean hormonal imbalances are impossible. Stress, diet, birth control use, and lifestyle factors can still affect your hormonal health.

The Menstrual Cycle: A Monthly Dance of Hormones

During your 20s, the menstrual cycle is typically regular, with the ebb and flow of **estrogen** and **progesterone** playing a pivotal role in reproductive health. At the start of each cycle, **follicle-stimulating hormone (FSH)** from the pituitary gland stimulates the growth of follicles in the ovaries. These follicles release **estrogen**, which prepares the uterine lining for a potential pregnancy. Ovulation occurs around mid-cycle when a surge in **luteinising hormone (LH)** causes an egg to be released.

After ovulation, the follicle transforms into the **corpus luteum**, which produces **progesterone**. Progesterone helps stabilise the uterine lining and supports early pregnancy if conception occurs. If no pregnancy happens, progesterone levels fall, leading to menstruation. This cyclical interplay ensures reproductive health, but it is also why women might experience PMS, cramping, or mood swings depending on the balance between estrogen and progesterone.

Testosterone: More Than Just a Male Hormone

Testosterone is commonly associated with men, but it plays a vital role in women's health, too. In your 20s, testosterone helps maintain muscle mass, bone strength, and libido. It is produced in small amounts by the ovaries and adrenal glands. Low levels of testosterone can result in fatigue, decreased libido, and reduced muscle tone.

Birth Control Pills and Hormonal Effects

Many women in their 20s use oral contraceptives to prevent pregnancy. However, it is essential to understand how these medications affect hormone levels. Birth control pills work by suppressing natural hormone production, particularly **ovulation**. The synthetic hormones in birth control replace the body's own production of estrogen and progesterone, often leading to side effects like mood changes, weight gain, or decreased libido.

Supporting Your Hormones in Your 20s

- **Exercise Regularly**: Physical activity helps regulate your cycle and supports testosterone levels. Strength training is particularly beneficial for bone and muscle health.

- **Eat Nutrient-Dense Foods**: Foods rich in **healthy fats** (like avocado, nuts, and olive oil) are essential for hormone production. **Leafy greens**, **fruits**, and **lean proteins** provide the necessary nutrients to support hormone balance.

- **Manage Stress**: Chronic stress elevates **cortisol**, which can disrupt the delicate balance of reproductive hormones and lower libido.

Case Study: Sarah's Skin Struggles and Hormonal Imbalances

Sarah, 25, always struggled with acne, which persisted into adulthood. After trying numerous skincare treatments with no success, Sarah learned that her acne was likely tied to hormonal fluctuations. Blood tests revealed elevated levels of **androgens**—male hormones like **testosterone** that can cause acne by increasing oil production in the skin. With the help of a hormonal balancing plan that included dietary changes, stress management, and a low-dose hormonal contraceptive, Sarah's skin began to clear up.

Your 30s: Fertility, Family, and Hormonal Fluctuations

The 30s often mark a busy decade for women. Many are advancing in their careers, starting families, or both. Hormone levels remain stable for most of this time, but toward the late 30s, women might begin to notice changes as the body starts transitioning toward perimenopause.

Fertility and Hormonal Shifts

In your early 30s, your reproductive hormones are still relatively stable, but by your mid to late 30s, **estrogen** and **progesterone** levels may begin to fluctuate, leading to changes in your menstrual cycle and possibly fertility. By age 35, women experience a natural decline in **ovarian reserve**, meaning the number and quality of eggs decrease.

During this decade, pregnancy can bring about the most significant hormonal changes. **Human chorionic gonadotropin (hCG)** is produced during pregnancy, leading to increased production of **estrogen** and **progesterone**. These hormones support the growing fetus and prepare the body for childbirth. Post-pregnancy, hormones gradually return to normal, but this transition can be challenging for some women, resulting in **postpartum depression** or **hormonal imbalances**.

Progesterone and Cortisol: A Delicate Balance

In your 30s, you might notice that stress impacts your menstrual cycle more than before. Chronic stress leads to elevated **cortisol** levels, which can deplete **progesterone** and disrupt your cycle. Progesterone is not only important for reproductive health but also for mood regulation. Low levels can cause irritability, anxiety, and insomnia.

Progesterone is also known as the "calming hormone" because it helps counterbalance the stimulating effects of estrogen. When progesterone levels drop, it can lead to **estrogen dominance**, a condition where estrogen levels remain high relative to progesterone. Estrogen dominance can cause **weight gain, bloating**, and **irregular periods**.

Supporting Your Hormones in Your 30s

- **Sleep Hygiene**: Sleep is critical for hormone regulation, especially **melatonin** and **cortisol**. Aim for 7-9 hours of sleep each night and maintain a consistent sleep-wake cycle.

- **Optimise Nutrition**: Include foods rich in **vitamin B6**, **magnesium**, and **zinc** to support **progesterone** production.

- **Exercise Mindfully**: Incorporating both **strength training** and **cardio** helps manage weight, reduce stress, and maintain healthy hormone levels. However, be mindful of over-exercising, which can elevate cortisol.

Case Study: Emily's Postpartum Journey

After her second pregnancy, Emily, 34, struggled with **low energy**, **mood swings**, and irregular periods. She visited her doctor, who identified **low progesterone levels,** likely caused by the demands of pregnancy and chronic stress. Emily's treatment plan included **bioidentical progesterone** therapy to restore balance, along with mindfulness practices like **yoga** and **meditation** to reduce cortisol. Within a few months, she noticed significant improvements in her mood and energy.

Your 40s: The Perimenopausal Transition

Your 40s mark the beginning of **perimenopause**, a natural transition phase before menopause. Perimenopause can last anywhere from 4 to 10 years, during which **estrogen** and **progesterone** levels become erratic, causing a wide range of symptoms.

What Happens During Perimenopause?

During perimenopause, the ovaries gradually produce less **estrogen** and **progesterone**, but hormone levels fluctuate unpredictably. You might have one month with heavy bleeding and intense PMS, followed by several months with light or skipped periods. These hormonal swings can trigger symptoms like **hot flushes, night sweats, mood swings, fatigue**, and **brain fog**.

Estrogen Dominance and Progesterone Deficiency

A key feature of perimenopause is **estrogen dominance**. With lower levels of **progesterone**, estrogen can become dominant, leading to symptoms like **bloating, weight gain, breast tenderness**, and **irritability**. Estrogen dominance also increases the risk of conditions like **fibroids** and **endometriosis**.

Progesterone plays an essential role in **balancing estrogen** and stabilising the uterine lining. During perimenopause, progesterone levels drop more quickly than estrogen, leaving estrogen unopposed. This can result in heavy or irregular periods and **premenstrual dysphoric disorder (PMDD)**—an intense form of PMS.

The Role of Testosterone During Perimenopause

While often overlooked, **testosterone** is also critical during perimenopause. As you age, testosterone levels gradually decline, leading to **decreased libido, muscle loss, fatigue**, and **mood changes**. Supporting healthy testosterone levels through lifestyle interventions or bioidentical testosterone therapy can help alleviate these symptoms.

Supporting Your Hormones in Your 40s

- **Consider BHRT**: **Bioidentical hormone replacement therapy (BHRT)** can help alleviate symptoms of estrogen dominance and progesterone deficiency. This therapy involves using hormones that are chemically identical to those your body naturally produces.

- **Boost Phytoestrogens**: Foods like **flaxseeds**, **soybeans**, and **chickpeas** contain phytoestrogens, which can mimic estrogen in the body and help balance hormone levels.

- **Stay Active**: Regular **weight-bearing exercise** helps maintain bone density and muscle mass, both of which are impacted by hormonal changes.

Case Study: Lisa's Perimenopause Struggles

At 45, Lisa noticed irregular periods, **severe mood swings**, and **trouble sleeping**. Her energy levels plummeted, and she found herself snapping at her family for no reason. After consulting her healthcare provider, Lisa learned that she was in **perimenopause**, with declining progesterone and fluctuating estrogen levels. Lisa began **bioidentical hormone replacement therapy**, focusing on **progesterone** and **testosterone**. She also adopted a **whole-food, plant-based diet** rich in phytoestrogens. Within six months, her symptoms had improved significantly, and she felt more in control of her emotions.

Your 50s and Beyond: Menopause and Post-Menopause

Most women reach **menopause** between the ages of 45 and 55. Menopause is defined as the absence of menstrual periods for 12 consecutive months. After menopause, **estrogen** and **progesterone** levels remain consistently low, and the body adapts to this new hormonal environment.

Menopause Symptoms

The most common symptoms during menopause include **hot flushes, night sweats, vaginal dryness, mood changes**, and **decreased bone density**. While these symptoms can be uncomfortable, they are manageable with the right lifestyle interventions and, in some cases, hormone therapy.

Hormonal Health Beyond Menopause

After menopause, the risk of **osteoporosis, heart disease**, and **cognitive decline** increases due to lower estrogen levels. Estrogen plays a protective role in maintaining **bone density, heart health**, and **brain function**. Post-menopausal women can benefit from focusing on **bone health** through **calcium, vitamin D**, and **weight-bearing exercise**. Hormone replacement therapy can also support healthy **cognitive function** and **cardiovascular health**.

Supporting Your Hormones in Your 50s and Beyond

- **Calcium and Vitamin D**: These nutrients are essential for bone health, especially after menopause when estrogen levels decline.

- **Healthy Fats**: Include omega-3 fatty acids from sources like **fish, flaxseeds**, and **walnuts** to support cardiovascular and brain health.

- **Stay Mentally Engaged**: Activities that challenge your brain, like puzzles, learning new skills, or social engagement, help maintain cognitive function.

Case Study: Susan's Menopausal Journey

At 55, Susan struggled with **hot flushes, joint pain**, and **vaginal dryness**. She also worried about her bone health, as her mother had suffered from osteoporosis. After discussing her options with her healthcare provider, Susan decided to start **hormone replacement therapy (HRT)** to alleviate her symptoms. She also focused on **strength training** and increased her intake of **calcium** and **vitamin**

D. Within six months, Susan's Hot flushes had reduced, her joints felt more flexible, and she was confident she was taking steps to protect her long-term health.

Conclusion: Embrace Every Decade

Every stage of life brings its own set of hormonal changes, but with the right strategies, you can thrive at any age. By understanding how your hormones evolve through the decades, you can take proactive steps to support your health, stay energetic, and age gracefully.

This extended version of Chapter 7 dives deep into the hormonal changes women experience through the decades, offering both scientific insights and practical advice. Each section includes specific hormonal details relevant to each age group, case studies to illustrate real-life scenarios and actionable strategies to support women's health at every stage of life.

Continual Hormonal Health: No Need to Stop If Well Monitored

One of the greatest misconceptions about hormone therapy and hormonal health is the idea that it is something that has an expiration date. In reality, with proper monitoring and personalised care, hormonal health can be maintained well into later years, supporting not just longevity but quality of life.

Hormones are dynamic, meaning their levels will naturally fluctuate and adjust with age, stress, and lifestyle. However, through regular monitoring and adjustments to your hormone therapy plan— whether it is through **bioidentical hormones**, nutritional support, or lifestyle changes—you can keep your body functioning optimally at every stage of life.

Working closely with a healthcare provider to track your hormone levels and adjust treatments as needed ensures that you stay in balance, avoiding potential side effects or imbalances. The key is **Personalisation**: there is no one-size-fits-all solution when it comes to hormones, and each woman's journey is unique.

A Lifelong Journey to Vitality

There is no need to stop optimising your hormones as you age. With consistent care and monitoring, hormone therapy can be a lifelong ally in your pursuit of well-being, vitality, and ageing gracefully. As long as your hormone levels are regularly reviewed, adjusted, and balanced, you can continue to enjoy the benefits—whether that is increased energy, improved mood, stronger bones, or mental clarity.

Remember, hormones are not just about solving menopausal symptoms. They are essential messengers that can support every aspect of your life. With the right approach, you can live younger, longer, and embrace vitality well into your later years. There is no need to slow down or stop living your best life—your hormones can help you keep thriving.

Summary: Navigating Hormonal Changes Through Every Decade

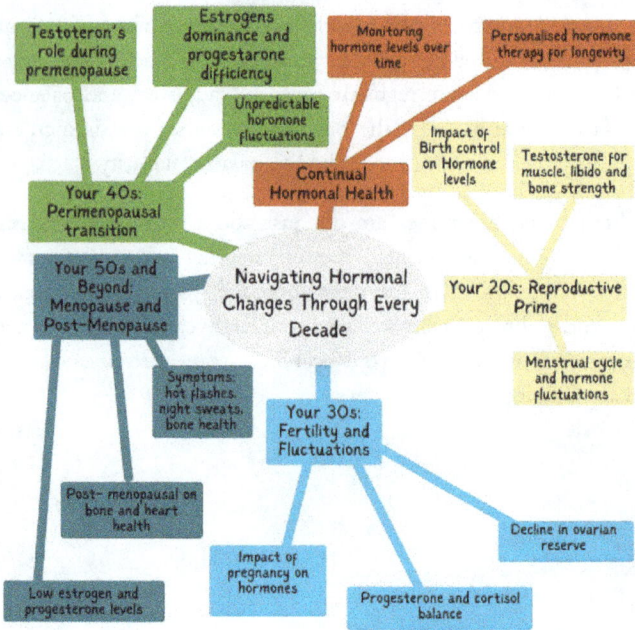

Testoteron's role during premenopause

Estrogens dominance and progestarone difficiency

Monitoring hormone levels over time

Personalised horomone therapy for longevity

Unpredictable hormone fluctuations

Impact of Birth control on Hormone levels

Continual Hormonal Health

Testosterone for muscle, libido and bone strength

Your 40s: Perimenopausal transition

Navigating Hormonal Changes Through Every Decade

Your 20s: Reproductive Prime

Your 50s and Beyond: Menopause and Post-Menopause

Menstrual cycle and hormone fluctuations

Symptoms: hot flashes, night sweats, bone health

Your 30s: Fertility and Fluctuations

Post- menopausal on bone and heart health

Decline in ovarian reserve

Impact of pregnancy on hormones

Low estrogen and progesterone levels

Progesterone and cortisol balance

Chapter 8
Hormones for Life – Personalising Your Long-Term Hormonal Health Plan

Hormones are vital to maintaining not just your reproductive health but also your overall well-being. Think of your body as a finely tuned race car. Each hormone functions like a critical component – the engine, transmission, tyres, and aerodynamics, all working together for optimal performance. In your younger years, the car runs smoothly, effortlessly speeding towards its goals. But with age, parts wear down, the engine might sputter, or the tyres lose their grip. Just like a race car needs regular maintenance and adjustments to stay competitive, your body requires personalised care to address hormonal shifts and maintain peak performance throughout life.

Why Personalisation Matters

There is no "one-size-fits-all" solution when it comes to hormones. Your body is unique, and what works for one person might not work for another. For instance, you might experience mood swings, fatigue, or weight changes due to hormonal shifts. At the same time, someone else might face different symptoms altogether. This is why creating a personalised hormone health plan is essential—it ensures you get precisely what your body needs.

Think of your hormones as "managers" overseeing different departments in a busy company. Estrogen, progesterone, and testosterone manage reproductive health, while cortisol and adrenaline handle stress responses. If one of these managers goes on vacation or becomes overwhelmed, the company (your body) does not run as smoothly. Personalising your hormonal health is like hiring extra support or reorganising responsibilities to keep things on track.

Building a Personalised Plan

The first step in building a long-term hormonal health plan is understanding your unique hormone profile. This typically involves comprehensive testing to assess your hormone levels and monitoring them regularly. Once you know what your levels are, you and your healthcare provider can design a plan that is tailored to your body's specific needs.

Your personalised plan might include:

- **Bioidentical Hormone Therapy (BHRT)**: These hormones are identical to those produced by your body, meaning they fit perfectly into your system and are less likely to cause side effects compared to synthetic hormones. BHRT is often adjusted to suit your body as it changes over time, ensuring you get the support you need without overloading your system.

- **Lifestyle Modifications**: Nutrition, exercise, and stress management play significant roles in maintaining hormonal balance. Healthy fats, like those found in avocados and nuts, support hormone production, while regular exercise helps regulate the whole system. Stress management techniques such as meditation can also help keep cortisol levels in check.

- **Supplements**: Nutritional deficiencies can throw your hormones out of balance. Ensuring you are getting enough magnesium, zinc, and vitamin D can help prevent imbalances and keep your hormone levels stable.

Hormone Monitoring: Regular Tune-Ups for Your Body

Hormones are dynamic, meaning they are constantly changing based on your life stage and lifestyle. Just like you would not drive a car for years without checking the oil or getting a tune-up, your hormones need regular check-ups too. Hormonal monitoring ensures that your levels remain balanced and that your treatment plan can be adjusted as needed.

Your hormonal health plan should be monitored every 3-6 months initially and once stabilised, at least once a year. This allows for adjustments based on your symptoms, life changes, and even external factors like stress or illness. For example, suppose you are going through a stressful period at work. In that case, your cortisol levels might spike, and that might require an adjustment in your hormone treatment.

Hormonal Needs Across the Decades

Your hormonal needs will evolve as you age, and your plan should adapt accordingly. Let us take a closer look at how your hormonal health changes through each life stage:

- **In Your 20s and 30s**: This is your peak reproductive time, and hormones like estrogen, progesterone, and testosterone are at their highest levels. Your hormonal plan will focus on keeping these hormones balanced to support fertility, mood, and metabolism. This is also a good time to check on your thyroid function, as it plays a role in metabolism and energy.

- **In Your 40s**: As you enter perimenopause (the transition to menopause), hormones can fluctuate, leading to symptoms like weight gain, mood swings, and changes in your menstrual cycle. A personalised hormonal plan, which may include BHRT, can help smooth out these fluctuations and support bone health, which can be impacted by decreasing estrogen levels.

- **In Your 50s and Beyond**: Once you reach menopause, your body produces less estrogen and progesterone, leading to potential symptoms like Hot flushes, night sweats, and bone density loss. In this stage, the focus of your hormonal plan will be on maintaining overall well-being, supporting bone health, and protecting against cognitive decline.

The Role of Bioidentical Hormones in Long-Term Health

Bioidentical hormones can be a crucial component of your long-term hormonal health plan. These hormones are molecularly identical to those your body naturally produces, which makes them easier for your body to process. Whether you are looking to balance mood, maintain energy levels, or protect your bones, BHRT can be personalised to fit your needs.

One of the biggest benefits of BHRT is its flexibility. Your doctor can start with a lower dose and adjust it as needed over time, ensuring that you are only getting what your body truly needs. As your hormone levels shift with age or life changes, your BHRT can be modified accordingly, keeping you balanced and healthy.

Think of BHRT like a custom-made suit—it is tailored specifically for you, and as your body changes, so can the fit.

Ongoing Adjustments: The Key to Success

Regular monitoring and adjustments are essential to ensure that your hormonal health plan continues to work for you throughout your life. Just like you adjust your wardrobe with the changing seasons, your hormonal plan should adapt to your body's evolving needs. Your doctor will check your levels periodically, adjusting your treatment to ensure optimal balance.

Hormones for Life: No Need to Stop if Well-Monitored

One common question about hormone therapy is whether there is a point when you should stop. The answer is no—if your hormones are monitored and adjusted correctly, you can continue using hormone therapy throughout your life. As long as you are regularly checking your levels, there is no reason to stop.

Hormones are essential for maintaining overall health and vitality. Stopping hormone therapy prematurely could lead to a resurgence of symptoms or put you at risk for conditions like osteoporosis. Think of hormone therapy as a tool that helps you maintain balance and stay healthy long-term, much like maintaining regular check-ups for your health in general.

Conclusion: Taking Charge of Your Hormonal Health for Life

Your hormones play a vital role in your overall health, and managing them is a lifelong process. By working with your healthcare provider to create a personalised hormone health plan, monitoring your levels regularly, and making necessary adjustments, you can ensure that your body stays balanced and healthy throughout every phase of life.

Summary: Navigating Hormonal Changes Through Every Decade

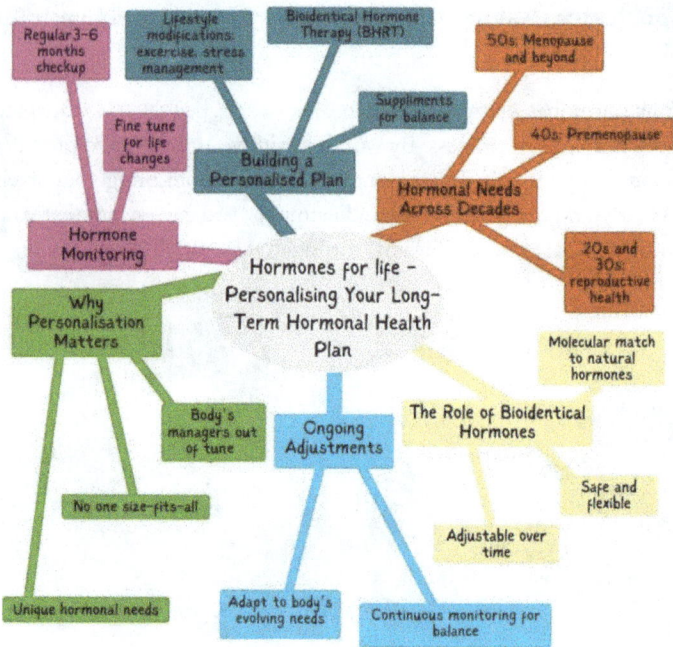

Regular 3-6 months checkup

Lifestyle modifications: exercise, stress management

Bioidentical Hormone Therapy (BHRT)

50s: Menopause and beyond

Fine tune for life changes

Suppliments for balance

40s: Premenopause

Building a Personalised Plan

Hormonal Needs Across Decades

Hormone Monitoring

Hormones for life – Personalising Your Long-Term Hormonal Health Plan

20s and 30s: reproductive health

Why Personalisation Matters

Molecular match to natural hormones

Body's managers out of tune

Ongoing Adjustments

The Role of Bioidentical Hormones

No one size-fits-all

Safe and flexible

Adjustable over time

Unique hormonal needs

Adapt to body's evolving needs

Continuous monitoring for balance

Chapter 9
Myths About Hormonal Safety – DHEA, Progesterone, Estradiol, Estriol, Pregnenolone, and Testosterone

When it comes to hormones, there are many myths and misconceptions, particularly around the safety of hormone replacement therapy. Hormonal imbalances can affect every aspect of a woman's life, and yet, many women avoid treatment because of these myths. This chapter will break down some of the most common myths about hormone safety and explain why, when properly monitored, hormones are both safe and beneficial.

Myth #1: Hormone Therapy Increases Cancer Risk

Perhaps the most persistent myth is that hormone therapy, particularly estrogen replacement, significantly increases the risk of cancer, especially breast cancer. This belief stems from early studies that suggested a connection between hormone replacement therapy (HRT) and breast cancer. However, the reality is more nuanced.

Estrogen-only therapy (used by women who have had a hysterectomy) has been shown to have a very low risk and, in some cases, may even reduce the risk of certain types of cancer. In women with intact uteri, combining estrogen with natural progesterone, rather than synthetic progestins, can lower risks considerably. Moreover, many women fear hormones without understanding that other lifestyle factors—such as obesity, smoking, and lack of exercise—pose a greater risk for cancer than hormone therapy itself.

Myth #2: DHEA Is Unsafe for Long-Term Use

DHEA (Dehydroepiandrosterone) is often misunderstood. Some believe that using DHEA over the long term can lead to dangerous side effects, such as an increased risk of cancer. In reality, DHEA is a naturally occurring hormone produced by the adrenal glands, and its levels decline as we age. Replenishing DHEA has been shown to have benefits, such as improving energy levels, boosting the immune system, and supporting sexual function.

When monitored by a healthcare provider, DHEA therapy is safe. It can be adjusted to suit your body's needs over time. Like all hormones, the key is regular monitoring to ensure balance.

Myth #3: Progesterone Causes Weight Gain

Many women are hesitant to use progesterone therapy because they fear it will cause weight gain. However, natural progesterone, unlike synthetic versions (progestins), is generally well-tolerated and does not cause weight gain. In fact, progesterone can help balance estrogen and prevent symptoms such as bloating and fluid retention, which are often associated with hormone imbalances.

Progesterone also plays a vital role in supporting sleep, reducing anxiety, and promoting bone health. When used in the right amounts, natural progesterone can be a powerful tool for improving overall well-being.

Myth #4: Estrogen Should Be Avoided After Menopause

Another common myth is that once a woman reaches menopause, she should avoid estrogen entirely to prevent health risks. However, estrogen plays a crucial role in protecting bone density, supporting heart health, and maintaining cognitive function.

After menopause, estrogen levels drop significantly, which can lead to symptoms such as hot flushes, mood swings, and osteoporosis. Using bioidentical estrogen, such as estradiol or estriol, can safely alleviate these symptoms and provide long-term health benefits.

Estriol, in particular, is a weaker estrogen that has been shown to provide protective effects without increasing cancer risks when used appropriately.

Myth #5: Pregnenolone Is not Important for Women

Pregnenolone is often overlooked in women's health discussions, but it plays a critical role in hormone production. Known as the "mother hormone," pregnenolone is the precursor to many other hormones, including progesterone, estrogen, and testosterone. Without enough pregnenolone, your body can not produce these vital hormones effectively.

Pregnenolone also supports cognitive function and helps manage stress. As we age, pregnenolone levels decline, which can lead to memory issues and decreased energy. Supplementing with pregnenolone, when properly monitored, can support overall hormonal balance and improve quality of life.

Myth #6: Testosterone Is Only for Men

Testosterone is often thought of as the "male hormone," but women need it too. Testosterone plays a critical role in maintaining muscle mass, energy levels, and libido in women. After menopause, testosterone levels often decline, leading to fatigue, loss of muscle strength, and decreased sexual desire.

Bioidentical testosterone therapy can safely restore these levels in women, helping to improve energy, mood, and overall vitality. Monitoring testosterone levels and adjusting treatment as needed ensures that women can enjoy the benefits without unwanted side effects.

Conclusion: Hormones Are Safe When Properly Monitored

The key to safe and effective hormone therapy is regular monitoring and working with a knowledgeable healthcare provider. Just like a well-tuned engine, your body needs the right balance of hormones to function optimally. When hormones are restored in the right amounts and carefully adjusted over time, they can be a powerful tool for maintaining health and well-being throughout life.

Do not let myths and misconceptions prevent you from exploring hormone therapy as a solution for managing the symptoms of hormonal imbalances. With the right guidance, hormones can be safely used to support energy, vitality, and longevity well into your later years.

Summary: Myths About Hormonal Safety – DHEA, Progesterone, Estradiol, Estriol, Pregnenolone, and Testosterone

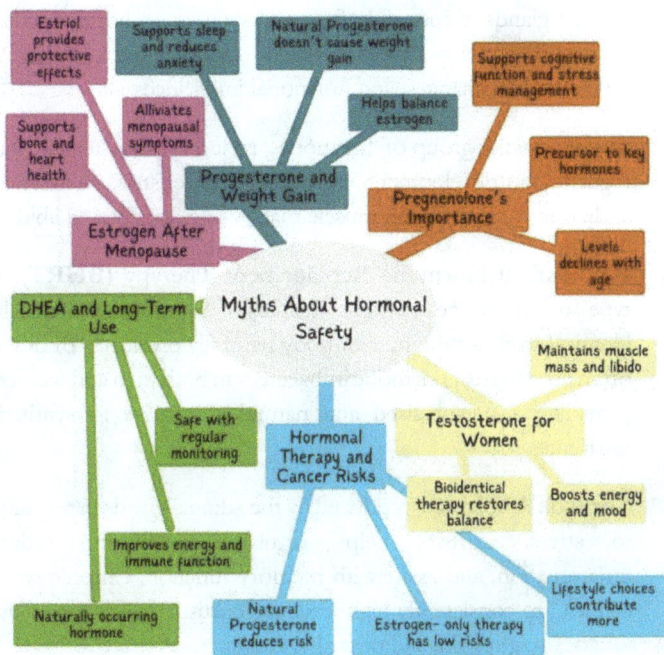

Glossary

1. **Adrenal Fatigue:** A term used to describe a condition where the adrenal glands, responsible for producing stress hormones like cortisol, become overworked due to chronic stress, leading to fatigue, mood changes, and hormonal imbalances.

2. **Androgens:** A group of hormones, including testosterone, that regulate the development of male characteristics. In women, androgens help maintain muscle mass, bone density, and libido.

3. **Bioidentical Hormone Replacement Therapy (BHRT):** A type of hormone therapy that uses hormones chemically identical to those the human body naturally produces. BHRT is often used to treat hormone imbalances in both men and women, providing a personalised and natural alternative to synthetic hormones.

4. **Cortisol:** A hormone produced by the adrenal glands in response to stress. Cortisol helps regulate metabolism, reduce inflammation, and assist with memory function. Chronic stress can lead to consistently high levels of cortisol, which may cause fatigue, weight gain, and other health issues.

5. **Dehydroepiandrosterone (DHEA):** A hormone produced by the adrenal glands, DHEA serves as a precursor to both estrogen and testosterone. Its levels naturally decline with age, and DHEA supplementation can support energy, mood, and immune function.

6. **Endocrine System:** The system of glands that produce and release hormones into the bloodstream. This includes the thyroid, adrenal, and pituitary glands, as well as the ovaries in women and testes in men. The endocrine system regulates metabolism, growth, reproduction, and stress response.

7. **Estrogen:** A group of hormones responsible for the development and regulation of the female reproductive system

and secondary sexual characteristics. Estrogen also plays a crucial role in maintaining bone health, skin elasticity, and cardiovascular function. The three main types are:

- **Estradiol (E2)**: The most potent form of estrogen, dominant during a woman's reproductive years.

- **Estriol (E3)**: A weaker form of estrogen, important during pregnancy and known for its protective role in breast health.

- **Estrone (E1)**: A weaker estrogen produced after menopause.

8. **Estrogen Dominance**: A condition where estrogen levels are higher relative to progesterone, leading to symptoms like weight gain, mood swings, bloating, and menstrual irregularities. Estrogen dominance can increase the risk of certain cancers if not properly balanced with progesterone.

9. **Follicle-Stimulating Hormone (FSH)**: A hormone produced by the pituitary gland that stimulates the growth of ovarian follicles (which house the eggs) in women and the production of sperm in men. FSH levels rise during perimenopause and menopause.

10. **Hormones:** Chemical messengers produced by glands in the endocrine system that regulate various functions in the body, including metabolism, growth, reproduction, mood, and energy levels.

11. **Hormone Replacement Therapy (HRT):** A treatment used to relieve symptoms of menopause by replacing hormones that the body no longer produces. HRT can include synthetic or natural hormones, such as estrogen and progesterone, to alleviate symptoms like Hot flushes, night sweats, and mood swings.

12. **Luteinising Hormone (LH):** A hormone produced by the pituitary gland that triggers ovulation in women and stimulates

the production of testosterone in men. High levels of LH can indicate that a woman is in perimenopause or menopause.

13. **Menopause:** The time in a woman's life when her menstrual cycles permanently stop, marking the end of reproductive ability. Menopause typically occurs between the ages of 45 and 55 and is characterised by a decline in estrogen and progesterone levels.

14. **Micronutrients:** Vitamins and minerals that are essential for hormone production and overall health. Examples include magnesium, zinc, and vitamin D. Deficiencies in micronutrients can lead to hormonal imbalances and other health issues.

15. **Osteoporosis:** A condition characterised by weakened bones, making them more prone to fractures. Declining estrogen levels during menopause can accelerate bone loss, making osteoporosis a common concern for postmenopausal women.

16. **Perimenopause:** The transition period leading up to menopause, during which hormone levels fluctuate, causing symptoms like irregular periods, mood swings, and Hot flushes. Perimenopause can last for several years before menopause officially begins.

17. **Pregnenolone:** Known as the "mother hormone," pregnenolone is a precursor to many other hormones, including progesterone, estrogen, and testosterone. It plays a crucial role in hormone balance and supports cognitive function and stress management.

18. **Progesterone:** A hormone that regulates the menstrual cycle and supports pregnancy by preparing the uterus for implantation of a fertilised egg. Progesterone also helps balance the effects of estrogen and plays a role in maintaining mood and sleep quality.

19. **Progestin:** A synthetic form of progesterone used in some hormone therapies and birth control pills. While effective in regulating menstrual cycles, progestins can carry more side effects compared to natural progesterone.

20. **Reproductive Years:** The period in a woman's life, typically between puberty and menopause, when she is capable of becoming pregnant. During this time, hormone levels, such as estrogen and progesterone, fluctuate to regulate the menstrual cycle and fertility.

21. **Sex Hormone Binding Globulin (SHBG):** A protein that binds to sex hormones, such as testosterone and estrogen, in the bloodstream. SHBG controls the amount of hormones that are available to the body's tissues, and high levels can reduce the amount of free testosterone or estrogen.

22. **Synthetic Hormones:** Labouratory-made hormones that are designed to mimic the hormones naturally produced by the body. While effective, synthetic hormones may carry more risks of side effects compared to bioidentical hormones.

23. **Testosterone:** Although primarily known as a male hormone, testosterone plays a vital role in women's health as well. It helps maintain muscle mass, libido, energy, and mood. Testosterone levels naturally decline with age and can be restored through hormone therapy.

24. **Thyroid Gland:** A butterfly-shaped gland located in the neck that produces hormones responsible for regulating metabolism, energy levels, and body temperature. Thyroid hormones include thyroxine (T4) and triiodothyronine (T3).

25. **Thyroid Stimulating Hormone (TSH):** A hormone produced by the pituitary gland that stimulates the thyroid gland to produce thyroid hormones. High levels of TSH can indicate an underactive thyroid (hypothyroidism), while low levels may indicate an overactive thyroid (hyperthyroidism).

26. **Triiodothyronine (T3):** The active form of thyroid hormone that regulates metabolism and energy production in the body. T3 is more potent than its precursor, thyroxine (T4), and plays a crucial role in maintaining a healthy metabolic rate.

27. **Vaginal Atrophy:** Thinning, drying, and inflammation of the vaginal walls due to decreased estrogen levels, often occurring during menopause. This can lead to discomfort, pain during intercourse, and an increased risk of urinary infections.

28. **Women's Health Initiative (WHI):** A long-term study initiated in the early 1990s to investigate the health risks and benefits of hormone replacement therapy in postmenopausal women. Some results of this study led to concerns about the safety of hormone therapy. However, newer research has clarified its benefits when used correctly.

References

1. Anderson, G. L., et al. "Effects of Estrogen Plus Progestin on Gynecologic Cancers and Associated Diagnostic Procedures: The Women's Health Initiative Randomized Trial." *JAMA*, vol. 290, no. 13, 2003, pp. 1739-1748.

2. Anisimov, V. N., et al. "The Role of Hormones in Ageing and Cancer." *Biogerontology*, vol. 3, no. 4, 2002, pp. 187-194.

3. Archer, D. F. "Tissue-Selective Estrogen Complexes for Postmenopausal Women." *Menopause*, vol. 15, no. 5, 2008, pp. 862-871.

4. Ayyar, V. S., et al. "Bioidentical Hormone Therapy: An Evolving Option for Women in Menopause." *International Journal of Women's Health*, vol. 11, 2019, pp. 221-230.

5. Barbieri, R. L. "The Endocrine Basis of Gynecologic Disorders." *Journal of Clinical Endocrinology and Metabolism*, vol. 90, no. 3, 2005, pp. 1296-1300.

6. Basaria, S., et al. "Testosterone Replacement Therapy and Cardiovascular Risk." *Journal of the American Medical Association*, vol. 310, no. 17, 2013, pp. 1829-1836.

7. Bhavnani, B. R., et al. "The Safety of Estrogen Therapy: A Risk-Benefit Analysis." *Endocrine Reviews*, vol. 27, no. 2, 2006, pp. 249-270.

8. Bianchi, V. E. "Testosterone's Effects on the Brain and Behavior in Elderly Men: Clinical Implications." *Frontiers in Endocrinology*, vol. 10, 2019, article 299.

9. Bianchi, V. E. "The Anti-Inflammatory Effects of Testosterone." *Journal of Endocrinological Investigation*, vol. 38, no. 7, 2015, pp. 759-763.

10. Bilezikian, J. P., et al. "Estrogen's Effects on Bone in Women." *Endocrine Reviews*, vol. 21, no. 4, 2000, pp. 307-317.

11. Boonyaratanakornkit, V., et al. "Estrogen Receptor Signaling Pathways in Human Diseases." *Journal of Steroid Biochemistry and Molecular Biology*, vol. 102, no. 1-5, 2006, pp. 113-119.

12. Boronat, A. C. "Thyroid Function and Bioidentical Hormones." *Journal of Thyroid Research*, vol. 2011, 2011, article 512498.

13. Bove, R. "Cognitive Function and Hormone Therapy in Menopause." *Current Opinion in Neurology*, vol. 33, no. 2, 2020, pp. 247-252.

14. Braam, L. A., et al. "Hormone Therapy and Cardiovascular Health: The Benefits and Risks." *Journal of Cardiovascular Medicine*, vol. 6, no. 4, 2005, pp. 233-241.

15. Brown, S., et al. "Bioidentical Hormone Therapy: A Review of the Evidence." *Obstetrics & Gynecology International*, vol. 2011, 2011, article 836135.

16. Burt, V. K., et al. "The Relationship Between Hormones and Depression." *Journal of Clinical Psychiatry*, vol. 65, 2004, pp. 28-33.

17. Cagnacci, A., et al. "Effects of Hormone Therapy on Sleep Quality in Menopausal Women." *Sleep Medicine Reviews*, vol. 23, 2015, pp. 20-27.

18. Chlebowski, R. T., et al. "Estrogen Plus Progestin and Breast Cancer Incidence and Mortality in Postmenopausal Women." *Journal of the American Medical Association*, vol. 304, no. 15, 2010, pp. 1684-1692.

19. Clark, S. A., et al. "The Role of Hormones in Muscle and Bone Health." *Clinical Endocrinology*, vol. 89, no. 3, 2018, pp. 235-245.

20. Davis, S. R., et al. "Menopause, Hormone Therapy and Women's Health." *Endocrine Reviews*, vol. 43, no. 2, 2022, pp. 211-233.

21. Dimitrakakis, C., et al. "Androgens and Breast Cancer in Women." *Endocrine-Related Cancer*, vol. 9, no. 3, 2002, pp. 207-214.

22. Dunn, P. K., et al. "Testosterone and Cognitive Function in Ageing Women." *Frontiers in Endocrinology*, vol. 11, 2020, article 142.

23. Eghlidi, D. B., et al. "Hormone Imbalances and Sleep Disturbances." *Endocrine Practice*, vol. 22, no. 10, 2016, pp. 1227-1238.

24. Faubion, S. S., et al. "Bioidentical Hormone Therapy: A Review of Safety and Efficacy." *Mayo Clinic Proceedings*, vol. 91, no. 4, 2016, pp. 453-464.

25. Fugh-Berman, A. "The Risks of Bioidentical Hormones." *International Journal of Health Services*, vol. 40, no. 1, 2010, pp. 77-89.

26. Gordon, J. L., et al. "The Role of Hormones in Mood and Anxiety Disorders." *Psychoneuroendocrinology*, vol. 53, 2015, pp. 85-100.

27. Grodstein, F., et al. "Hormone Therapy and Cardiovascular Disease: Results from the Nurses' Health Study." *Annals of Internal Medicine*, vol. 135, no. 10, 2001, pp. 753-763.

28. Guaschino, S., et al. "Role of Estrogens in Cognitive Function and Neuroprotection." *Maturitas*, vol. 74, no. 4, 2013, pp. 313-320.

29. Healy, D. L., et al. "Progesterone and Progestins in Women's Health." *Maturitas*, vol. 32, no. 3, 1999, pp. 143-152.

30. Hildreth, K. L., et al. "Role of Estrogen in Preventing Cardiovascular Disease." *Endocrine Reviews*, vol. 32, no. 3, 2011, pp. 456-482.

31. Hodis, H. N., et al. "Testosterone Replacement Therapy in Women: Is it Time?" *Menopause*, vol. 24, no. 5, 2017, pp. 497-500.

32. Holtorf, K. "The Bioidentical Hormone Debate: Are Bioidentical Hormones Safer or More Efficacious?" *Postgraduate Medicine*, vol. 121, no. 1, 2009, pp. 73-85.

33. Howell, L. P., et al. "The Effect of Estrogen and Progesterone on the Breast and Cancer Risk." *Endocrine Reviews*, vol. 21, no. 4, 2000, pp. 307-317.

34. Hunt, K., et al. "Effects of Hormone Therapy on Skin and Hair in Women." *Journal of the American Academy of Dermatology*, vol. 75, no. 2, 2016, pp. 291-300.

35. Jenkins, M. R., et al. "Estrogen and Bone Health in Postmenopausal Women." *International Journal of Women's Health*, vol. 4, 2012, pp. 341-348.

36. Kaunitz, A. M., et al. "Bioidentical Hormones for Menopause Management: Evidence and Implications." *Climacteric*, vol. 23, no. 2, 2020, pp. 114-121.

37. Klinge, C. M. "Estrogen Regulation of Mitochondrial Function and Biogenesis." *Journal of Endocrinology*, vol. 205, no. 1, 2010, pp. 1-12.

38. Lobo, R. A., et al. "Hormone Therapy and the Cardiovascular System." *New England Journal of Medicine*, vol. 365, no. 2, 2011, pp. 147-156.

39. Longcope, C. "Androgen and Estrogen Dynamics in Women." *Endocrine Reviews*, vol. 12, no. 1, 1991, pp. 101-117.

40. MacLennan, A. H., et al. "Hormone Therapy in Perimenopause: A Review of Safety and Benefits." *Cochrane Database of Systematic Reviews*, 2001, article CD003924.

41. Martin, K. A., et al. "Clinical Benefits of Bioidentical Hormone Replacement Therapy." *Fertility and Sterility*, vol. 75, no. 4, 2009, pp. 523-530.

42. Maturana, M. A., et al. "Hormones and the Brain: Evidence from Menopausal Women." *Journal of Neuroendocrinology*, vol. 28, no. 9, 2016, article e12440.

43. Nappi, R. E., et al. "Impact of Estrogen on Mood, Sleep, and Mental Health in Women." *Climacteric*, vol. 19, no. 1, 2016, pp. 41-46.

44. Nelson, H. D., et al. "Postmenopausal Hormone Therapy and Breast Cancer Risk." *Journal of the American Medical Association*, vol. 288, no. 3, 2002, pp. 321-333.

45. Panay, N., et al. "Progesterone and Its Role in Hormone Replacement Therapy." *Maturitas*, vol. 47, no. 4, 2004, pp. 269-275.

46. Pines, A. "Cardiovascular Benefits and Risks of Bioidentical Hormones." *Journal of Women's Health*, vol. 22, no. 10, 2013, pp. 864-870.

47. Pines, A. "Osteoporosis Prevention with Bioidentical Hormones." *Journal of Bone and Mineral Research*, vol. 27, no. 5, 2012, pp. 1107-1114.

48. Pinkerton, J. V., et al. "Hormone Therapy and Health-Related Quality of Life." *Climacteric*, vol. 18, no. 2, 2015, pp. 172-180.

49. Reed, S. D., et al. "Bioidentical Hormones and Endometrial Safety." *Menopause*, vol. 16, no. 3, 2009, pp. 380-389.

50. Ritenbaugh, C., et al. "Risks and Benefits of Hormone Therapy." *Journal of Women's Health*, vol. 22, no. 4, 2013, pp. 288-297.

51. Santen, R. J., et al. "Management of Menopausal Symptoms: Estrogen and Beyond." *Endocrinology and Metabolism Clinics of North America*, vol. 50, no. 2, 2021, pp. 243-272.

52. Sarrel, P. M. "Hormone Therapy for Cardiovascular and Cognitive Function in Women." *Endocrine Reviews*, vol. 32, no. 3, 2011, pp. 237-254.

53. Schmidt, P. J., et al. "Mood, Cognition, and Hormones: The Critical Role of the Menopausal Transition." *Menopause*, vol. 12, no. 6, 2005, pp. 564-576.

54. Schneider, H. P. G., et al. "The Role of Hormones in Ageing and Longevity." *Journal of Endocrinology*, vol. 192, no. 3, 2007, pp. 387-397.

55. Stuenkel, C. A. "The Role of Progesterone in Hormone Therapy." *Journal of Clinical Endocrinology and Metabolism*, vol. 94, no. 8, 2009, pp. 2546-2549.

56. Tsai, S. A., et al. "Testosterone Therapy and Risk of Cardiovascular Events." *Journal of Clinical Endocrinology and Metabolism*, vol. 100, no. 8, 2015, pp. 3479-3492.

57. Usadi, R. S., et al. "Hormonal Control of Female Reproduction." *Journal of Reproductive Medicine*, vol. 65, no. 3, 2017, pp. 234-244.

58. Utian, W. H. "Menopausal Hormone Therapy and Long-Term Risks." *Cochrane Database of Systematic Reviews*, 2016, article CD004143.

59. Warren, M. P., et al. "Hormonal Regulation of Muscle and Bone Health in Women." *Endocrine Reviews*, vol. 24, no. 2, 2003, pp. 243-264.

60. Zivadinov, R., et al. "Hormonal Influences on Cognition and Neurological Function." *Menopause*, vol. 18, no. 1, 2011, pp. 61-69.